HOW I DID IT

A FITNESS NERD'S GUIDE TO LOSING FAT & GAINING LEAN MUSCLE

NATE CLARK

FITNRD
An imprint of **SNAZZY CO.**

This book is intended for informational purposes only and does not constitute medical advice. You should not rely on this information as a substitute for, nor does it replace, professional medical advice, diagnosis, or treatment. You should consult your doctor before starting any fitness, diet, or similar program, including those set forth in this book. This book is intended for healthy adults 18 years and older. This book is not intended for those in poor health or with preexisting health conditions. If you choose to follow any advice in this book, then you do so voluntarily and assume all related risks.

Results may vary.

HOW I DID IT:
A Fitness Nerd's Guide to Losing Fat and Gaining Lean Muscle

FIRST EDITION

Designed by Jules Klein

Library of Congress Control Number: 2019955951

Identifiers: ISBN 978-1-951876-01-2 (hardback) | 978-1-951876-03-6 (paperback) | 978-1-951876-00-5 (epub) | 978-1-951876-04-3 (kindle) | 978-1-951876-05-0 (audiobook)

For Cary. Never stop trying.

CONTENTS

Foreword   vii

Introduction   ix

PART ONE: THIS IS ALL IN YOUR HEAD   1

1. The Hard Truth   3
2. Goal-Setting   9
3. Start Obsessing   17
4. Eyes on the Prize   25
5. So, You're Not a Kid Anymore?   33
6. Overcoming Setbacks   37

PART TWO: FOOD IS 90% OF YOUR PROBLEM   43

7. There Is Only One Way to Lose Fat   45
8. Find Your Starting Point   55
9. Caloric Expenditure   67
10. Calculating Your Deficit   73
11. Carbs & Proteins & Fats   87
12. Finding the Right Macronutrient Balance   101
13. The Macro/Deficit Split for Fat Loss   115
14. Bulking vs. Cutting   123
15. Eating Clean   129
16. Foods I Avoid   137
17. To Cheat or Not to Cheat...   151

PART THREE: STRENGTH TRAINING   159

18. Strength Training Is Your Best Weapon   161
19. How to Track Your Gains   171

20. Compound Exercises vs. Isolation Exercises   179

21. Strength, Hypertrophy, or Endurance?   187

22. Check Your Form!   197

23. The Mind–Muscle Connection   205

24. Tempo & Rest   211

25. Stretching & Mobility Work   217

26. How Many Days per Week?   223

PART FOUR: CARDIO   231

27. The Real Purpose of Cardio   233

28. Cardio Is Not the Best Way to Lose Fat   239

29. HIIT It!   247

30. Walk It Off   253

PART FIVE: OTHER CONSIDERATIONS   257

31. The Only Fitness Supplements I Use   259

32. Go the Fuck to Sleep   273

33. Group Fitness   277

34. Gym Pet Peeves   283

THE PLANS   287

Putting It All Together   289

3-Day Split   291

4-Day Split   295

5-Day Split   299

Preferred Exercises   303

Grocery Shopping List   307

Acknowledgments   311

Notes   313

Index   321

About the Author   329

FOREWORD

Well, he did it! Then he undid it. Then he did it again! (And then he wrote a book about it.) What I've learned from watching Nate's fitness journey is that the rules to achieving fitness are relatively easy to follow. It's merely a matter of deciding to apply them every day.

In our 10 years together I've seen Nate go from his fattest to his fittest—from finding empty pints of convenience store ice cream hidden in the outside trash to packing snack bags of plain chicken and raw spinach. He went from being tired all the time to jumping out of bed at 5 a.m. to write in his journal and head to the gym.

I'm so proud that Nate's hard work has paid off and that he is sharing what he's learned along the way with the world (or at least you) through this book. Especially because it hasn't been easy—it took a lot of self-reflection, hard work, and above all else, a commitment to change poor habits. Also, I'd offer it took a supportive partner who would make sure that every restaurant had a healthy option for him (even if that option was ignored in favor of a burger and fries); a patient partner who could sit in silence for two minutes at the end of every meal so Nate could "enter his food" into his nutrition app; and a confident partner who tolerates the throngs of "Insta-fans" messaging him after a particularly thirsty progress pic on Instagram (eye-roll).

Nate's health kick inspired my own. We cook most of our meals at home, we shop for healthy groceries, and we go for long walks after dinner most nights. And I'm glad for it because I've realized how important it is to me to model a healthy lifestyle for our young son. (But, if our son ends up rebelling with pizza, cakes, and milkshakes, at least he'll have this book and some old photos of his hot dad and me to inspire him to change course.)

Regardless of your own aspirations, I wish you the best of luck on your journey to fitness and health. Surround yourself with supportive people, hold yourself accountable, and trust that if you "follow the math," as Nate says, you will achieve your goals. I know it's possible because I watched him do it.

Also, know that it took Nate many attempts to get there. I've heard him say "one last piece of cake" followed by "that was a mistake" more times than I can count. Just keep trying. This book contains all the tools you need to make it happen.

Happy reading, healthy eating, and good working out!

- ALLEN LOEB, NATE'S HUSBAND

INTRODUCTION

I used to be fat. I was a fat child, a fat teenager, and a fat adult. When I was a kid, my cousins called me "the frog" because my belly made me look like a toad. I swam with my shirt on until I was 25.

When I started high school, my family doctor told me I'd "probably be fat" for the rest of my life. I carried that with me into adulthood. I can still hear him taunting me. He convinced me that I would always struggle to lose weight. He made me believe I would never be fit. That fitness was impossible for me. He set me up for defeat.

I still think of myself as a fat kid. Some days I hesitate before I take my shirt off, even though I have no reason to. Looking back now, I realize he was a shitty doctor. His assumptions about my body defined me and caused many failed attempts to get in shape.

THE YO-YO EFFECT, a.k.a. "THE WEIGHT-LOSS ROLLER COASTER"

I rode the weight-loss roller coaster for most of my life. Maybe you have, too.

First, I'd get fed up with how my body looked—and how crappy I felt. I'd remember that doctor, and I'd get mad enough to make a change.

I would seek out the newest, most hyped, *guaranteed-to-change-your-body!* fitness program and I'd dive into it full force. I'd obsess about burning more calories, and I'd spend all my free time exercising.

I'd eat protein bars for breakfast, lunch, and dinner most days. I lived on the treadmill; I'd do more cardio than any sane person has time to do. Then I'd inhale a pint of ice cream—in my car, in secret—assuming I'd burn off those calories the next day.

And then I'd start to lose a little weight and begin to feel better about myself! *Hooray!* Unfortunately, I'd also be exhausted, lonely, and bloated, thanks to all the protein bars and ice cream.

After a few weeks my initial excitement would wane. Running for hours every week would become untenable. I'd get busy with other things (like living my life), so I'd take a break from the treadmill. And then I'd eventually stop exercising altogether, but I'd continue to eat the ice cream and the protein bars.

After a few more weeks, I'd discover that I'd regained any weight I'd lost and then some. I'd be frustrated and angry at myself, and I'd decide to do something about it again. "I'll stick with it this time!" I'd say to myself.

But I didn't, of course. **Because I liked to ride the weight-loss roller coaster.** But not really.

I repeated this cycle for decades. Losing weight, regaining the weight, trying to lose it again. Every attempt seemed more difficult than the last. Seriously, I've tried so many gimmicks to lose fat:

- I ran 50 miles a week on treadmills, staring at CNBC, running on a road to nowhere.
- I gave up meat for 12 years.
- I tried Atkins… and ended up eating raw butter out of my fridge.
- I tried CrossFit and got all banged up.
- I hired personal trainers and paid them thousands of dollars.
- I tried P90X videos and stained my carpets with puddles of sweat.
- I tried everything. Except for the obvious thing.

Between the ages of 21 and 35, I bought all the equipment. I bought the Ab Roller. I bought the boots that let me hang upside down for crunches. I bought countless pairs of running shoes and running watches and heart rate straps. I spent a small fortune on a fancy bicycle that I rode from San Francisco to Los Angeles. I bought it all.

None of it worked.

This is a photo of me at the beginning of 2014. My body fat was close to 30%, which the World Health Organization qualifies as "obese."

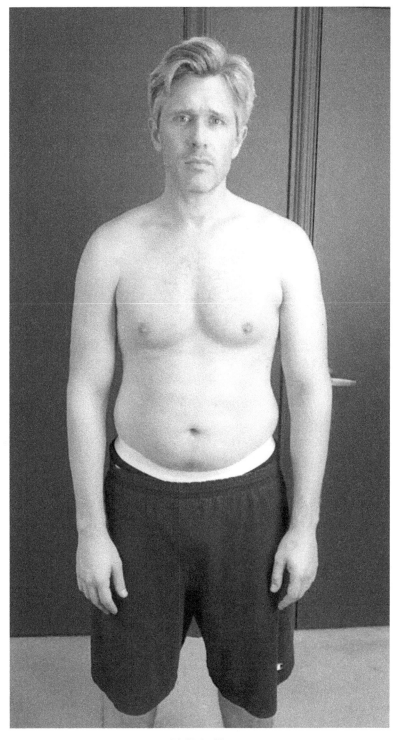

My "Before" Pic

I'm embarrassed by that photo, but my embarrassment goes well beyond the way I looked in the mirror. I'm embarrassed by how I felt—both physically and emotionally—and by my inability to fix the problem.

I felt tired all the time, so I would eat sugary and fatty foods to feel energized, then I would crash. I did this over and over again every day. Bags of potato chips. Swedish Fish. Every damn kind of protein bar you can imagine. The farts were outrageous.

More than anything, I felt guilty. I knew I was abusing my body, and I was ashamed of myself.

WHY I WROTE THIS BOOK

I wrote this book to share with you how I finally stepped off the weight-loss roller coaster and transformed my body. I hope the lessons I've learned inspire you to chase your own goals. I'm sure you've tried lots of fat-loss tactics, too. Maybe some even worked for a while, but they never got you where you really wanted to be. Or maybe you're stuck right now and you don't know how to break out of your current rut.

Let me begin by confessing something: *I'm super self-conscious about writing this book.* I'm not a personal trainer or a fitness professional—I'm a writer and filmmaker. I'm an average guy with a husband and a toddler. I'm not a bodybuilder. I'm not trying to be a "fitness guru." I'm not trying to sell you supplements or anything else.

I wrote this book because people kept asking me how I did it, and there was too much info to share it all in a casual conversation. I wrote it all down in my spare time because I want to show you how a regular guy like me stays in shape. I also want to differentiate science from hype, because I've read so much bullshit advice about fitness, and I want to clear the air about a few things.

The following photo is me after I lost 31 pounds of fat and added almost 10 pounds of muscle. I'm 40 years old and I'm in the best shape of my life. I never thought I'd look or feel this great. I thought it was impossible.

Last summer I was on vacation, walking along the beach, and a 20-something-year-old woman yelled out to me, "Hey, do you swim?" I assumed she was asking me if the ocean was safe to swim in, so I said, "Sure, there are a few rocks, but I think it's safe."

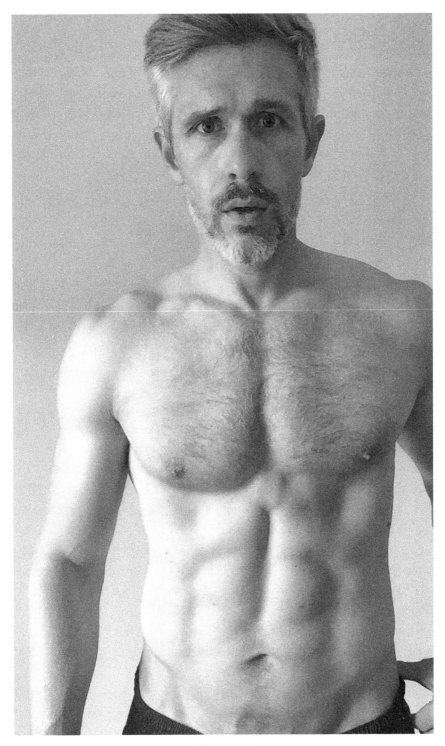

My "After" Pic

Then she said, "No. I mean, do *you* swim? What did you do to get that body?" I just… I couldn't believe it. Nobody had ever asked me anything like that before in my life. Not bad for a 40-year-old desk jockey.

Then more people started asking me the same things: What kind of workouts do you do? What do you eat? What *don't* you eat? Friends, strangers in elevators, random people kept asking. Eventually, enough people were curious that I decided to write this book. Because I wish someone had given me this information 20 years ago. I'm sharing my experience so that maybe you too will have a stranger ask you, "How did you do it?"

WHAT'S IN THIS BOOK?

This book is full of stuff you already know, even if you've never thought about it before. It's information your body instinctively understands. Your body will react naturally to this information as soon as you allow it to do so.

This book covers my current approaches to diet and exercise, and how I learned to ignore the never-ending stream of bullshit fitness products people try to sell me. Most importantly, I share the state of mind I maintain to accomplish my goals.

The fitness industry is mired in convoluted advice and strategies that confuse and obscure simple truths about fat loss. I wrote a book that walks you through the most vital concepts *you need to know* in order to transform your body. Some concepts may seem too simple and easy, but those are the areas you've probably neglected. Losing fat is so much more straightforward than the industry purports it to be. Gaining muscle is slightly more challenging, but it relies on all of the same mathematical truths.

I've organized this book as a reverse pyramid. Topics in this book flow from "essential" to "less important." The most vital concepts come first, and each subsequent chapter is less crucial than the previous chapter. Make no mistake: everything in this book merits your attention. But the tools in each chapter become progressively less imperative as the book moves forward. (It ends with a chapter about gym etiquette, which, let's be honest, you don't *need* to follow in order to get in shape.)

Also, a warning: I repeat myself throughout this book. *I repeat myself throughout this book.* Maybe more than I should. Sorry, not sorry. When I repeat a concept, it's because *I think it deserves to be repeated.* Repetition builds familiarity, which leads to better results.

ESSENTIAL

YOUR STATE OF MIND

CALORIES & MACROS

STRENGTH TRAINING

CARDIOVASCULAR
EXERCISE

EVERYTHING
ELSE

LESS IMPORTANT

IS THIS BOOK FOR YOU?

I wrote this book for people like me:

- If you struggle to lose fat, this book is for *you*.

- If you don't know how to gain muscle, this book is for *you*.

- If you're unhappy with your body but you're afraid there isn't anything you can do about it, this book is for *you*.

- If you've been going to the gym for a while but you haven't noticed a significant difference in how you look and feel, this book is for *you*.

- If you are confused by the seemingly infinite and contradictory fitness advice people keep barking at you, this book is *definitely for you.*

- If you're just trying to lose that last 10 pounds or reach single-digit body fat, this book is for *you too.*

- If you are *any* of the people I've just described, then you should stick around.

Yes, This Book Is for You

You want to lose fat. You want that lean, muscular body you've always dreamed of. You want to be energized and powerful, and you want to feel confident when you're naked.

Cool. You can have all of those things. **Get excited about transforming your body into the ideal body you've always wanted but never thought you could achieve.** You *are* capable of achieving it, and I'll tell you how. It will happen naturally, and much quicker than you expect.

But this book is not just for you.

It's also a reminder to myself, in case I forget again.

PART ONE:

THIS IS ALL IN YOUR HEAD

CHAPTER 1

THE HARD TRUTH

No man is more unhappy than he who never faces
adversity. For he is not permitted to prove himself.

SENECA

WE ARE FAT

In my late 30s my body fat percentage averaged between 27% and 30%. I was technically obese according to standards set by the National Institutes of Health (NIH).[1]

This isn't the most sensitive way to say this, and it might not even be popular opinion today, but I'm going to say it anyway:

Most of us are too fat.

I know that sounds harsh, but the data backs me up. According to an analysis by the Centers for Disease Control and Prevention (CDC), the average American man—at 5 feet, 9.25 inches tall—weighed 196 pounds in 2014. That's 15 pounds heavier than the average American man weighed in 1996.[2] The average American woman's weight increased by 17 pounds over the same period.

If that doesn't scare you, how about this? Researchers at the NIH assert that, in the US, as many as 91% of adults and 69% of children are "overfat."[3]

What does it mean to be overfat? Writing for Frontiers in Public Health, authors Philip B. Maffetone, Ivan Rivera-Dominguez, and Paul B. Laursen describe people who are overfat as those "who exhibit metabolic health impairments associated with excess fat mass relative to lean body mass."[4] Being overfat means we have too much fat relative to the amount of lean tissue, which includes muscle, organs, and bone. It indicates the amount of fat we carry is disproportionate to our body, not to someone else's body. It's more specific than words like "overweight" and holds less of a negative connotation than terms like "obese."

SIDE NOTE: The words we use to describe our bodies have a major impact on how we treat ourselves and each other. The article I mentioned above notes that by choosing "accurate, useful, and unintimidating terminology regarding abnormal body fat conditions," we increase awareness around the epidemic. Consider using the term "overfat" instead of "obese."

And yet despite having a clinical term that defines 91% of American adults, we're still reluctant to accept the fact that most of us are too fat. We often shy away from recognizing our fatness because too many of us are afraid to acknowledge it in our own lives. I've read several recent articles in popular magazines and newspapers attempting to sugarcoat these statistics, despite the overwhelming data proving that Americans are getting fatter. Many writers undermine the accuracy of the data seemingly for fear of fat-shaming readers. Some people even claim that carrying excess fat doesn't necessarily indicate greater health risks, despite overwhelming evidence to the contrary. Data charted for the past 40 years shows a correlation between increasing body fat among Western cultures and increases in several pathologies:

- There was a 45% increase in the prevalence of metabolic syndrome* among US adults ages 18 and up between 1988 and 2012.[5]

- Obesity is an independent risk factor for cardiovascular disease,[6] which now affects 48% of US adults.[7]

---

* Metabolic syndrome is a combination of the following conditions: increased blood pressure, high blood sugar, excess android fat, and high cholesterol. Collectively, these symptoms drastically increase the likelihood of stroke, heart disease, and type 2 diabetes.

- The Institute for Alternative Futures predicts a 54% increase in the total number of Americans with diabetes between the years 2015 and 2030.[8]

We can't ignore the problem any longer. We shouldn't disregard the fact that the majority of Americans are overfat solely because people are too afraid to confront the truth. We can't continue to destroy our bodies for the sake of not hurting people's feelings. Instead of avoiding the truth, we all need to accept it and collectively seek solutions to the problem.

WHY DID THIS HAPPEN?

Most of us already know *how* we got so much fatter than the generations before us. We know we eat out too much, and that portion sizes have blown up in recent decades. We know that healthy foods, like vegetables and fruits, seem to cost way more than the unhealthy options. The less healthy options are also faster and more accessible to many communities. And we know the industrial food supply chain prioritizes profit over nutrition. The list goes on.

But *why* did we allow all of this to happen? Why are we spectators watching ourselves get fatter and not seeming to care?

It's because an honest self-assessment of our health requires courage and humility. It's scary to confront uncomfortable truths about our bodies. We're afraid of the truth, so we've normalized "fat." We tolerate our excess body fat even in the face of dangerous consequences. We don't consider ourselves to be overfat, although the evidence says we are. What's more, we disregard that we feel like crap, that we're tired all the time, and that our fatness might impact more than just our appearance.

Collective Acceptance

I believe we've accepted our collective fatness as a reaction to the unrealistic standards of beauty set by the media. We're berated by photos of overly skinny, unsustainably muscular, impossibly lean men and women in commercials, television shows, movies, and ads plastered across every available screen. Our minds are flooded by imagery suggesting that we aren't thin enough, jacked enough, or beautiful enough. Profit-driven businesses set unattainable standards for beauty and health in an effort to sell us stuff.

These supposedly "ideal" bodies are ridiculous and, ultimately, dishonest.

We react to these false standards with equally false compromises. Knowing (at least subconsciously) that these standards are impossible, we have repositioned personal standards for beauty at an equally impractical distance from average, just in the opposite direction. The media shows us unreasonably skinny people, so we push back by increasing our tolerance for being unreasonably overfat. We excuse our shortcomings as if to reinforce the impossibility of media standards. Instead of accepting the media's absurd references for fitness, we tell ourselves (and our kids) that it's okay to be overfat because we need to "love ourselves."

Of course we need to love ourselves! But loving yourself doesn't preclude you from acknowledging that you are overfat. Bodies come in all shapes and sizes. You can love your body while also keeping your body fat percentage down at a healthy level. Further, the best way to love yourself is to honor your body by treating it well. It's the only body you've got.

Honoring your body *does not* mean accepting someone else's standard of fitness or beauty. **It means becoming the best version of yourself that you can imagine. Feeling good when you breathe, when you walk, when you get out of bed in the morning.**

I'm not telling you what I think your ideal body fat percentage should be. Only a doctor (or the NIH, the CDC, and so on) has the right to call you "unhealthy."

But you know how you feel. If you are reading this book, you are probably unhappy with your body, for one reason or another. If that's how you feel, it's time to own it.

Mindless Eating

I think you know when the food you eat is good—that is, good for your body. You know in your heart when food fuels your amazing, creative, energetic, vibrant existence on this planet. You might also know when you eat certain foods because you are addicted to them. We're all getting better at discerning which foods make us feel good and which foods make us feel crappy.

However, you might not realize *how much* you eat or if that amount supports your daily activity level. You might be unaware of how much food you truly need, and you might not notice that you consume two or three times that amount on a daily basis. Overeating even the healthiest foods will still cause you to gain fat. And, unfortunately, most of us eat way more than we need to.

The Food and Agriculture Organization of the United Nations indicated that the average amount of calories consumed by American adults (as of 2016) was 3,757 calories a day.[9] That's a 30% increase in average calories consumed in 1961 (2,880 calories).[10] That's also 29% more calories than the worldwide average of 2,904.[11] They warn that this increase is the primary cause of the ~~obesity~~ overfat epidemic we are experiencing.

Most of us consume more food than we need to because we aren't paying attention. It's become too easy to overeat, especially when the food industry wants to convince us to eat more (i.e., buy more). But we need to pay attention! We need to start appreciating how many calories our bodies actually require, and then eat according to those requirements. We need to eat *mindfully* and let our bodies guide us.

For all the people who keep asking me how I lost all that fat, here's the short answer:

I stopped overeating.

CHAPTER 2

GOAL-SETTING

Greatness is not achieved when the result is reached,
but rather long before that, when an individual
chooses to do the things that he knows he needs to do.

BRIAN P. MORAN & MICHAEL LENNINGTON,
The 12 Week Year

Don't rush your expectations. Anticipating results is the first mistake you can make in your pursuit of any fitness plan. The fitness industry thrives on false expectations and the promise of instant miracles, but it's time for you to ignore all of that. Urgency will sabotage your goals. I know impatience was a prime contributing factor in my failed previous attempts to get fit. I spent too much energy expecting results instead of focusing on the task at hand, today, right now.

I got over that, and so should you. When it comes to reaching your goals, the only moment that matters is *right now.*

This very moment.

Not yesterday. Not five minutes ago.

Not tomorrow. Not next January.

And definitely not *after* you've achieved your goals.

GREATNESS HAPPENS NOW

The results you crave are a culmination of many smaller decisions you make continually. Every moment of your life is an opportunity to take a small step toward realizing your larger goal. Instead of anticipating future results or searching for answers in the past, you must focus on the step you can take at this moment in time. Because you only have control over the action you take *right now.*

> **Greatness happens NOW, not after you notice the results of your greatness. Results are merely an acknowledgment of the greatness you've already achieved.**

Small Goals

You can achieve any significant goal by concentrating on smaller goals throughout the day. To succeed, you need to break apart your big goal into tiny goals, and then commit to accomplishing those goals as often as possible. The bigger your long-term goal, the smaller the goals you'll need to define. Devote yourself to goals you can achieve *right now,* and you will eventually reach your bigger goal *without any additional effort.*

Big Goals Are Hard

When you focus on the big, seemingly impossible goals, you grow impatient when they don't happen quickly enough. You feel defeated if you slip along the way because failure reinforces the idea that your big goal is *impossible.*

Let's say you want to lose 50 pounds this year. That goal probably seems huge to you. Maybe even impossible. Truthfully, losing 50 pounds is no easy task for anyone, regardless of their fitness level or body composition. But try reframing that huge goal this way: *I want to lose one pound this week.*

Does that seem impossible? One pound is a small number. It might even seem easy. If it doesn't feel easy, how about shaving that goal down to this: *I want to lose half a pound this week.* Now you have a smaller goal that seems much easier to achieve.

> **The secret to getting fit is to keep whittling down your big goals into smaller ones you can achieve <u>today</u>.**

Small Goals Are "Easy"

Do you have a habit of eating a muffin every day for breakfast? If your small goal is to skip that muffin—and opt for something healthier—you can achieve that goal *right now*.

Today's small goals might be as straightforward as getting to the gym or hitting my macros. They might be as effortless as committing to skipping dessert at a dinner party, or as simple as walking to the post office instead of driving there.

Small goals might seem trivial to you, but they do add up. I've seen my body change in ways I never thought possible because I committed myself to small goals every day.

Plus, small wins are a reason to celebrate, and celebrating motivates you to succeed again tomorrow. That's how I feel every time I skip dessert or forgo the latte or eat my apple without peanut butter. *I feel proud of myself.* I feel greatness at that moment because I have achieved a small goal on the path to my larger goals. I enjoy accomplishing those tiny goals every day. Every small goal I achieve motivates me to keep at it and to achieve more goals the next day.

Small goals are easy to achieve, and I feel great immediately after I check them off my list. That's much more rewarding than waiting six months from now to feel proud when I recognize that I've accomplished a huge goal.

Celebrate Now, Not Later

I often see people reward themselves for achieving long-term fitness goals by engaging in the exact behavior they were avoiding in the first place (e.g., eating an entire pizza after a month of dieting). They're missing the point.

Of course you want to celebrate when you achieve a long-term goal. Maybe you should "treat yo'self" by buying a new bathing suit or planning a romantic trip with your partner. But why would you celebrate all that hard work by purposefully trying to unravel it with bad behavior?

That's the joy of setting small daily goals: **achieving a small goal feels like a reward in and of itself.** When I accomplish a small goal—like making the decision to skip dessert—I'm proud of myself then. That's my reward. I feel good about the decision I made at that moment. I don't need to wait until next month to feel like I achieved something.

Likewise, I'm not going to reward myself for skipping dessert by eating a different dessert five minutes later. That would be crazy. It's easier to see why that sort of reward doesn't make sense when I'm focused on the small action I took five minutes ago, instead of something I achieved over the course of two months. Rewarding yourself with food *never* makes sense.

Are You Rolling Your Eyes?

It's okay if you are. I used to be just like you. No joke. I used to look at a doughnut and think, "I can eat this, it doesn't matter." And then I'd stare at a picture of some ripped dude in a fitness magazine while I ate my doughnut, wishing I knew his secrets, shaking my fists at the sky, cursing my bad genes.

Then I'd get depressed and reach for a second doughnut.

That's how they get you to buy more doughnuts.

But now I've changed how I think about my goals. Instead of focusing on that fitness model and his rock-hard abs (see: "impossible" goals) I've shifted my focus to the doughnut. I know that if I cut that doughnut out of my day today, I take a step toward seeing my own abs. I just have to say no to that one friggin' doughnut, at this moment, right now. That's it! Before I know it, those missing doughnuts snowball into achieving my "impossible" goal.

Thinking this way is the key to achieving the body you want. If you are still rolling your eyes, then you aren't ready to achieve your goals.

DEFINING YOUR SMALL GOALS

You may have tried similar goal-setting techniques before, but it's possible that your goals weren't small enough. Here's how I define a small goal:

> A small goal is <u>actionable</u>, meaning you
> can achieve it with a single action.

The larger the goal, the more distant success seems to be, because bigger goals require *multiple* steps. However, you achieve a small goal immediately after the action is completed.

To put this into action, you must reframe the decisions you make each day as small goals on the path to health and wellness. Create a series of small goals and a system to implement these goals for the week ahead. Choose goals that are manageable and inspire confidence. The more prepared you are, the more likely you are to achieve these small goals as challenges arise.

You can also refine your small goals on the fly. Set small goals each day when you wake up. Set a small goal when you sit down to order lunch. Set small goals when you walk in the gym. Set a small goal when you're headed to the grocery store and tempted to buy a pint of ice cream.

Here are a few bigger goals that can be reframed into smaller ones:

BIGGER GOAL	SMALLER GOAL
I will lose 25 pounds.	I will skip my morning doughnut today.
I will grow my biceps two inches this year.	I will add one more set to each of my bicep exercises today.
I will drink a gallon of water today.	I will drink 16 ounces of water this morning.
I will walk 10,000 steps today.	I will get up from my desk and walk 500 steps this hour.

Continue to break bigger goals down into smaller ones. *A truly small goal is one you can accomplish with the least amount of effort.* Big goals take time, and they lack noticeable results in the short term. Instead of being frustrated while waiting to achieve your long-term goals, focus on goals you can accomplish every day, every hour, every minute... *right now.*

Example of a Small Goal in Action

I'm getting ahead of myself, but I want to provide you with an example here. Let's stick with the goal I mentioned earlier: to lose a half-pound of fat this week. (You might now consider this a *medium*-size goal.)

A half-pound of fat is merely a clump of potential energy waiting to be burned. We measure that energy in calories, another unit of energy you are probably more familiar with. A half-pound of fat is equal to 1,750 calories. If you want to lose half a pound a week, then 1,750 / 7 days = 250 calories per day. (Much more info about calories coming up ahead.)

To lose half a pound of fat this week, you need to cut 250 calories each day, all else equal. Here's a list of foods in the 200–300 calorie range:

- A Snickers Original Bar[12]
- A dozen dried apricots
- Twenty Nacho Cheese DORITOS[13]
- One serving of peanut butter
- A tall (12-ounce) Caffè Mocha from Starbucks[14]

This is a brief list of the countless ways you could cut 250 calories from your diet today. (Hint: all foods come in 250-calorie sizes.) So, how about setting the following small, daily goal: *I will cut 250 calories from my diet today.* You can achieve that goal by simply skipping *one* of those foods listed above! All else equal, if you achieve that goal every day this week, you will also achieve your larger goal without even considering it.

I talk about calories in much greater detail in Part Two of this book, but for now, use this example to shift your mindset toward prioritizing small goals over bigger ones.

ASSEMBLE THE DATA

Record your successes and failures every day, and then review the data to ensure that your small goals yield the results you expect. There are many ways to track your small goals, and I cover my preferred methods throughout this book. You might use a notebook or a spreadsheet or one of the myriad apps available for smartphones if that's your thing. Regardless of how you do it, make a plan to document these goals continuously.

Every second week, use this data to review how well you did in the context of your bigger goal. Building on our example of losing half a pound of fat per week, I suggest you evaluate how many days you were able to cut that 250-calorie item. (Seven out of seven? Four out of seven?) Take a look at your average weight for the week and compare how it changed against your rate of successfully achieving small goals. You might consider waiting to review the data until you've been at it for three weeks, a month, or longer, in order to gather a larger data set. Larger data sets yield a more reliable assessment of your progress.

Assess the Data

Sometimes you will fail to achieve your small goals. (That doughnut is calling your name like, "Hey, girl, hey!") That's okay! There is another small goal out there with your name on it. If you only achieved your small goal three days out of seven, you might consider an even smaller goal. Instead of trying to skip the muffin every day, shoot for skipping it on Monday, Wednesday, and Friday.

Don't be hard on yourself if you struggled to achieve these small goals. Research shows that kids (and therefore likely adults) who are fat-shamed only gain more weight.[15] I'm confident that fat-shaming *yourself* can be an even worse deterrent to achieving your dreams. Don't judge yourself and don't sweat the small failures. If you didn't achieve your small goals, reassess and set *new* goals that you're more likely to achieve. No goal is too small.

Likewise, if you skipped that muffin seven out of seven days and you think you're ready for more, try adding another small goal to your routine. Maybe you can cut another 250 calories a day from someplace else. Or maybe you are ready for even more ambitious daily goals.

The important thing is that you avoid frustration. Frustration kills progress. Reconsider your small daily goals if you aren't satisfied at the two-week mark, but no sooner than that. Don't be too eager. Don't get frustrated, and don't give up. Always set small goals you can crush, and challenge yourself within your limits. I promise you that these small goals will add up, but only if you keep at them. Focus on this moment right now, and everything will begin to change for you in ways you never thought possible.

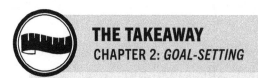

THE TAKEAWAY
CHAPTER 2: *GOAL-SETTING*

Greatness happens now, not after you notice the results of your hard work. The results are merely an acknowledgment of the greatness you've already achieved.

Don't focus on your long-term goal. Instead, **set small, actionable goals you can accomplish every day.** These small goals have a cumulative effect; you will eventually achieve your big goals without any extra effort.

Small goals are <u>actionable</u>, meaning you achieve them with a single action. Planning to skip your morning doughnut, go for a walk, or squeeze out one more set of biceps curls are all examples of small goals.

Small goals add up. Choose your small goals wisely and celebrate your achievements every day.

Record your small goal successes and failures every day. Use this data to periodically evaluate your fat loss and muscle-building progress against your consistency in accomplishing small goals. Bi-weekly or monthly is often enough. If you aren't satisfied with your progress, reconsider your small goals. If you failed to achieve your small goals consistently, pick easier goals and check back in another two weeks.

CHAPTER 3

START OBSESSING

You have power over your mind – not outside events.
Realize this, and you will find strength.

MARCUS AURELIUS

AN OBSESSIVE MINDSET

You need to *obsess* about your goals in order to achieve them. What do I mean by "obsess"? No, I'm not advocating mental illness. Chill out. When I say you need to obsess about your goals, I mean *you need to keep those goals top of mind at all times*. Set an intention, and then consider it throughout the day. Be mindful:

- If you decide to eat at the Chinese restaurant, think about how that impacts your daily caloric goal.

- If you decide to stay up late to watch a movie on Netflix, consider how you'll feel working out tomorrow.

- If you travel for work, investigate the equipment at the hotel gym before you go. Plan your workouts that week to accommodate your change of venue.

By obsessing about your greater intentions, you constantly evaluate your choices based on their contribution to your goals, big and small. Make an effort to continuously reflect on the things that matter most to you, and consider how every little decision you make impacts your results. Balance your decisions against your small goals. You make better choices when you contemplate how those choices affect your goals.

- It's easy to skip a second beer at the bar if you think about how it will impact the pursuit of your ideal body fat percentage.

- It's easy to shut your phone off before bed if you think about how a good night's sleep will impact your morning workout.

- It's easy to remember to order the salad dressing on the side if you think about maintaining a caloric deficit for the day.

Obsess about the things you want to achieve, and one day you will wake up surprised to realize that you have already achieved them.

Have You Heard of *The Secret*?

In case you haven't, or if you forgot, here's a quick refresher. It's a program for achieving your dreams through positive visualization. There is more to it than that, but that's *The Secret* in a nutshell. It's a philosophy that suggests:

You are what you think about.

They call it "the Law of Attraction," and it says that the things you pay attention to are the things the universe brings you. *If you think about the things you want, they will materialize in your life as if by magic.*

If you focus on gratitude for the things you have, you will attract more things to be grateful for. Similarly, if you worry about the things you fear, so too will those things manifest in your life in one way or another.

The people behind *The Secret* have written several books about this philosophy. They host widely attended seminars, and they even made a movie about it. There are a lot of details and specifics, and the book is worth reading. But, in my estimation, *The Secret* boils down to one single idea: *I am what I envision myself to be.*

If I envision myself succeeding, I will succeed. Likewise, if I envision myself failing, I will fail. If I think about how impossible a big goal seems, I guarantee that the goal remains impossible. This is yet another reason I focus on small daily goals I'm confident I can achieve.

Yeah, sure, whatever… The first time I heard this philosophy I thought it was bullshit too. "You mean, I can have whatever I want just by *thinking* about it?" It seems like there are simple ways to test the limits of this philosophy. For instance, I am thinking about levitating out of my chair right now, so hard that my brain hurts, but it ain't happening.

Using the "I can't fly" litmus test, I previously discarded *The Secret* as New Age woo-woo. I assumed it was an excuse people used to avoid putting in the work needed to achieve their goals. I forgot about *The Secret* for years. And then something happened. **I realized I was doing *The Secret* by accident, and it was working.**

After years of half-assed attempts to get in shape, I began to *obsess* about getting the results I wanted. I diligently tracked the data I needed to track—diet, exercise, sleep, and so on—and I *concentrated* on losing fat and gaining muscle. I thought about what I was eating and how I was progressing, all day long. I began to plan my food in the morning and pay attention to every single thing I ate, asking myself, *Does this serve my goals? Am I really hungry for this?*

I kept my small goals at the top of my mind all day, and then I began to see results like never before.

> *You become what you think about most. But you*
> *also attract what you think about most.*
>
> JOHN ASSARAF

POSITIVE VISUALIZATION

The Secret isn't a magic spell to solve your problems or a mystical way to achieve your dreams. It is, in essence, an exercise in positive visualization. When we visualize reaching our goals, we train our brain to see the impossible as probable.

Use positive visualization to imagine how your life will be when you achieve your big goals:

- Envision the smile on your face as someone asks you how you got in such great shape.

- See yourself in the mirror with the body of your dreams.
- Imagine yourself moving through a room with energy and confidence.

You should also use positive visualization to picture yourself achieving small, daily goals:

- Visualize yourself saying "no" to that doughnut later this morning, and smiling when you've achieved that goal.
- Visualize yourself walking into the gym tomorrow morning at 6 a.m.
- Visualize yourself blasting through that bench press set, and then resting after your hard work.

Fill your day with visions like this. **Constant positive visualization tethers you to your goals.** If you visualize yourself succeeding, then you will instinctively take action toward that success. Positive visualization maintains a mind-body connection; see it in your mind, and your body will do it.

You Are What You Think About

Positive visualization changed the way I exercise. I've been working out for my entire adult life. Despite years of exercise, I have never been as fit as I am right now. And I'm 40 years old! I achieved this level of fitness by obsessively visualizing it all day, even when I didn't realize that's what I was doing at the time. I am obsessed with being in the best shape I can be, and that's why I am in shape.

To be clear, I'm not obsessive in a clinical way. I think about other things besides fitness. (I've got a toddler at home, and he is my most important responsibility!) But when it comes to my *personal* goals, fitness comes first.

I've also noticed that I've become more productive in other areas of my life as I've become more mindful of my fitness goal. Likewise, being fit and feeling good about myself boosts my mood—and I know my family likes me better when I am happy!

Someone else might choose to say they are "constantly mindful" instead of calling themselves obsessive. Yes, you want to remain mindful throughout the day, but mindfulness might connote passivity. Obsessing amplifies mindfulness. I'm more than merely *aware* of my goals; I continuously *engage* in achieving them by visualizing the results I want. Obsession makes an impact.

If the word "obsession" sounds unhealthy to you, then use whatever word you want. The point is that you must think about your goals at all times. If you visualize success, you will act in ways that support it. Even if these thoughts are passing blips in a sea of thoughts throughout a busy day, they inspire action and ensure that every decision you make gets filtered through the lens of your goal.

> Obsession inspires action. When you obsess about something, you inevitably act on that obsession in one way or another.

Make the Time

You "don't have time" to obsess about fitness, right? Wrong. You might think you're too busy to make fitness your primary focus. I get it. My life is complicated too. I'm lucky in some regards because I set my own work schedule, but I also have a toddler and pets and a house with plumbing that breaks and three full-time jobs (for real)… so yeah, I'm busy too.

Still, I achieve my goals because I obsess about them. Why? Because for me (and most everyone else, I bet), **physical health is integral to everything else I do.** When I'm healthy, I have more energy, better focus, and I am happier. That last one is crucial:

> Being fit makes me happy, and when I'm happy, my "problems" disappear.

It's all about perspective. So how do I make time to obsess about fitness, even when my schedule becomes unreasonably complicated? I keep visualizing success even when life gets messy. I *see* myself making the time to achieve the small goals I want to achieve. I *envision* myself going to the gym in the early morning if that's the only time I'll be able to go. I *envision* myself prepping a healthy dinner for my family hours ahead of time, so we aren't tempted to order takeout at the last minute. I *envision* peak physical fitness throughout the day, and it remains my top priority.

When I obsess about it, I avoid making excuses when I'm presented with life's little challenges. No matter what comes up, I manage to find the time to act on my goals, sometimes in surprising ways. **The universe makes it possible for me to exercise and eat healthy** *because I want it to.*

That's the blueprint for achieving your goals, fitness-related or otherwise. It's not enough to simply want something without obsessing about it. There is no value in only trying to reach your goals when it's convenient. In my experience, life is rarely convenient for more than an hour or two.

Stay focused on your goals. All day. Every day. Visualize them. Write them down. Record the data as you work toward reaching them. Here are a few more suggestions of ways to obsess about fitness throughout your day:

- **Journal about your goals in the morning.** Write them down. There is no pressure to write well. Just write in a stream of consciousness about the things you want, and think about the small goals you are going to achieve today.

- **Check-in with your food journal throughout the day—** every time you eat something, at the very least. (More info on food journaling later, I promise.)

- **Take progress photos and put them in places you'll see them, like your phone's home screen.** Remind yourself of *why* you're on this path. (Pictures can be a powerful tool, so be careful not to judge yourself or compare yourself to others. Keep it positive and aspire to be the best YOU that you can be.)

- **Curate music playlists for upcoming workouts** (if music helps keep you motivated) and share them with friends. Search for new songs and envision how they will keep you energized at the gym.

- **Use your lunch break to read about muscle groups and how they work.** The more you know, the better you'll do in the gym.

- **Listen to a podcast about fitness or nutrition on your way home from work.**

The possibilities are endless. When you obsess over your goal you discover how even the most routine choices you make can impact your success. The essential point is to *keep thinking about your goals.*

I've come to believe that this is the secret to getting fit. Or ripped. Or jacked. Or whatever healthy means to you. It's also the key to landing your dream job. Or making 10 million dollars. Or achieving anything else you want. (Just remember that people are not something to obsess about. Please don't go stalking anyone. And please, *please* don't tell anyone I told you to obsess about them, because I did not!)

If you really want something, you will think about it constantly. If you think about it, you will act on it. And if you act on it, *it will happen.*

THINK ABOUT YOUR GOAL.
KEEP IT AT THE TOP OF YOUR MIND ALL DAY.

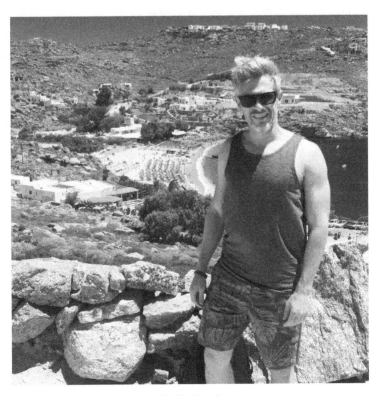

Do You Swim?

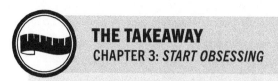

THE TAKEAWAY
CHAPTER 3: *START OBSESSING*

Check out *The Secret*. It's a philosophy proposing that you are what you think about. It's not magical thinking; it's a technique for positive visualization.

Envisioning success creates a connection between your mind and your body. When you imagine yourself succeeding, you convince your brain of the reality of that success. When your brain is convinced, it forces your body to act in support of that reality. Positive visualization leads to action, which in turn leads to achievement.

The solution for achieving your toughest goal is to **obsess about it.** Your goal—and the action steps you put in place to accomplish it—should be top of mind at all times.

Obsessing isn't compulsive when you consciously choose to obsess. You don't need to sacrifice your attention to other things, like family or work, in order to obsess about fitness. Obsessing just means that you filter all of your actions through a check-in about your goals. For instance, ask yourself: *How will this decision impact my goal to lose 50 pounds this year?*

Seek out new habits and activities that will help you keep your goal top of mind throughout the day. For example, spend your lunch break researching muscle groups, making an exercise playlist, or planning your next workout.

CHAPTER 4

EYES ON THE PRIZE

There is nothing noble in being superior to some other man. True nobility is being superior to your previous self.

SENECA

YOU ARE YOUR ONLY COMPETITION

Here's another tip about your mindset before I dive into the nuts and bolts of fat loss and muscle growth. As you begin this transformation into the ideal version of yourself, no matter what happens, no matter how excited or disappointed or frustrated or massively successful you are, remember this:

This is your journey, not anyone else's.

Everyone is different. Each person has different genes, different life circumstances, and different obligations. Unfortunately, that cliché about the grass always being greener is true. It's human nature to become jealous after watching what your neighbor is doing over there in the corner.

So, *don't watch your neighbor.*

Please concentrate on your grass, capisce? Solve *your* problems. Keep your eyes on the prize, and don't worry about how anyone else is doing on their fat-loss or strength-training journey.

Pics Will Deceive You

Pictures of beautiful people show up everywhere. I see so many pics of fitness professionals with extremely lean physiques and gigantic muscles, often performing Ninja Warrior–style acrobatics. None of those pics accurately portray how messy, weird, and imperfect we all are.

TV and magazine ads bombard us with pics of twenty-something models who spend nearly 100% of their waking life in the gym. Professional stylists paint and pluck them, and then the pics are butchered in Photoshop.

I would guess that 99% of professional fitness photos are fake in one way or another. I'm not only talking about using computers to wipe away love handles or add shadowy definition to abs—both of which are standard practice. I'm talking about the three weeks of starvation and dehydration that the model did leading up to the shoot. That's not real life! **It's impossible to live in a constant state of photo-readiness.** Don't believe any of it.

Social Media Is Not Real Life Either

We also have to see carefully crafted social media posts by friends and family. Everyone self-promoting, and every post strategically intended to provoke an emotional response in others. To make you feel something about the person who posted it, instead of focusing on how *you feel* today.

We live in odd times. I am inundated with Instagram posts, Facebook messages, and a seemingly endless stream of people yelling, "Look at me! Look at me!" on social media platforms galore. I assume it's the same for you too.

Everywhere I look, I see people with their heads bowed, their eyes glued to their smartphones. I watch fingers tapping and flicking and flipping through… pictures of other humans. Many of them strangers. Photos of other humans doing things, eating things, being places.

Why do we spend so much time watching other people live their lives? *I'm guilty of it too.*

In turn, viewing all this social media pressures us to advertise our best selves to keep up with everyone else. We try very hard to show the world how fantastic our lives are, editing those photos with filters and brushes that distort the truth. We spend all of this time on self-promotion instead of self-reflection, creating a vicious cycle whereby everyone thinks more about everyone else than they do about their own objectives.

This is how excessive exposure to social media can tank your fitness goals. We see these "best self" advertisements posted by others, and we compare ourselves to them, even though they aren't an accurate portrait of reality. Often these posts make us feel "less than" because we don't meet their unrealistic expectations of success. They have the same effect as mass media.

People (and businesses) share these posts with their own agenda in mind, and often that agenda is to make you jealous so that you'll buy something or "follow" someone. Their objective is to provoke an emotional response in you, and you have no control over their tactics for doing so.

Just remember that nobody is born with the perfectly sculpted body they just posted on Instagram, and nobody looks like that 100% of the time. We all have bad days. We all struggle. Every perfect fitness pic you see is a combination of hard work, good lighting, and lies… and you will never know how much of each.

You Probably Compare Yourself to Others Subconsciously

You might not think you compare yourself to other people, but you probably do it more than you realize you do. You might not always be conscious of it, but it's happening subconsciously.

Continuous, conscious self-reflection is a challenging habit to master. I'm certainly not there yet. When I scroll through Instagram I usually forget that I'm thinking more about the lives of strangers than I am thinking about my own life. When I see someone attractive or wealthy and I think, "That looks great—they're lucky," I subconsciously compare myself to them. Or at least, I'm comparing myself to the image they're presenting.

Well-crafted images—especially those used in marketing—are *engineered* to force you, the viewer, into subconsciously creating a values story around that image. A values story is a narrative describing the people in the image: what they are doing, how they got there, and what *values* led them to the moment when the photo was taken.

Good marketers can skillfully suggest a values story and plop it into your head before you even realize what's happening. They aim to align their product with your values so that you will in turn identify their product as something that supports your ideals, and then buy whatever they're selling. All of this happens instantaneously.

For example, take a look at the following photo of a man on a cliff:

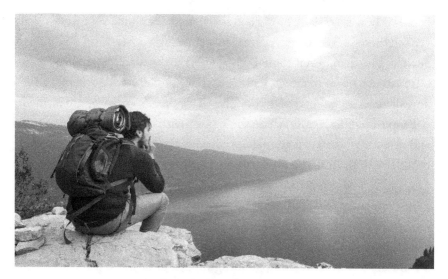

Credit: frankie's/Shutterstock.com

First question: what did you expect when I said "take a look at this photo of a man on a cliff"? Did you anticipate something terrible or dangerous?

But this is a picture of a man at ease. When you see this picture, you tell yourself a values story about the man you see, and you imagine a context (i.e., the reasons) for why he's there. Here's the story I see:

There's a man. He's alone. He's wearing a pack, so he's been traveling or hiking. He's high up, and he probably worked very hard to get to the top of this peak. He's lucky. He's looking out over a calm sea. He seems peaceful. I wish I felt like that. I wish I was traveling. ***I wish I had this guy's life****... and so on.*

That's a values story. I've ascribed values to the person I see in this image, and I am comparing them to my own. I admire some of the things I've fantasized about this guy, and I envy his imaginary accomplishments. The advertisers reflect back at me both what I want to see and what they want me to see.

Truthfully, I don't know anything about the guy in this photo other than what I see. I don't even know his name. Everything else I made up in my own brain. He could have been dropped on the edge of this cliff by a helicopter, or he could be sitting in front of a green screen on a Hollywood soundstage. He could be dying of cancer. *I have no clue.* And yet, the story I imagined when I described the picture a minute ago is the story I wanted to tell myself. It's an aspirational story. I see my values, my hopes, my dreams reflected back at me.

And we all do this thousands of times every day. Probably most times we look at a picture, and especially when we see a picture of someone who has something we want. So, even if you don't think you compare yourself to others, you probably do it subconsciously. You add a values story to the images you like based on the values you aspire to, and then you instantly compare that story to your current state of being.

The only way to avoid making that comparison is to remain conscious when you look at these images. Remember that every image has a purpose—a story to tell. Stay mindful of your own goals and objectives, not the values story someone else is selling you.

If you want to succeed at a plan to lose fat, gain muscle, and transform your body, you need to focus on *your own body*. Concentrate on yourself and your goals, and fight the temptation to be distracted by how other people look and feel. There is no time for comparison to other people's bodies. Someone else's body is entirely, totally, 100% unattainable for you. What do I mean by that?

You can't be anyone else. You are you.

If you want to see bigger muscles or a slimmer waist, stand in the mirror and envision yourself looking like that. Instead of looking at other people's bodies for inspiration, I suggest you examine where you are and then imagine yourself as you want to be. There is power in that sort of positive visualization!

If you decide to look at photos for fitness inspiration, do so sparingly and take them with a grain of salt. Remember that these images aren't true to life. Look for photos that show honesty, commitment, and real tips for improving your workouts. You don't need to obsess over someone else's physical appearance. Keep *your* goals top of mind and remember that nothing anyone posts online is the whole picture.

PAY NO MIND IRL, EITHER

While we're on the subject of comparing ourselves to others, it helps to remember that this also applies in the real world, too. Especially in the gym.

It's easy to feel intimidated by strangers in the gym: guys benching hundreds of pounds, muscles bulging, looking fit and much more experienced than you; ladies who can run an eight-minute mile then step off the treadmill, glistening, and head into a kickboxing class without blinking.

Don't sweat it. Comparing yourself to other people in the gym will screw up your path to success by creating false expectations for your own journey.

There will always be some guy at the gym benching 320 pounds. He'll be grunting, dropping the bar loudly to the floor as if to scream, "Hey, everybody! Look at my pecs! Aren't they AWESOME?!"

Don't let him distract you. Don't let him intimidate you. You aren't here to be like him; you are here to be like *you*. And even though you aren't as strong as him today, remember that everyone—even that grunter—started somewhere. He wasn't born with those giant pecs.

Even if you are an experienced lifter, there will always be someone with more experience than you. I guarantee it.

Focus on Yourself IRL

- You need to lift an amount of weight that works for *you* for each exercise you plan to do today.

- You need to eat a lunch that meets *your* goals, not the lunch your co-worker or boss has in mind today.

- You need to run or walk at a treadmill speed that works for *you*, not the guy who is cranking on the machine next to you.

It Doesn't Matter How Much They Lift

Most days, I do biceps curls with 10-pound dumbbells. I'm not kidding. There might come a day that I need to drop the weight even more than that.

So what?

The number on the dumbbell, machine, or plate only matters when I compare it to other numbers in my personal history of lifting. I don't worry about the numbers on the weights that anyone else is lifting. I don't let it get me down if I can't add another plate this week. And I don't get intimidated by anyone else's progress. I track my progress like it's my religion, and I ignore what others do in the gym. *I pretend like they aren't there.*

Lift What You Can

If you need to perform an exercise with a naked bar (i.e., without plates), then that's where you need to be today. If you are experienced but you want to push yourself further, don't use anyone else's expectations to determine how much further you can go, or how much weight to add to the bar today.

Keep your eyes on the prize. If your eyes start to wander to the guy or gal on the bench next to you, move to a bench in a different room.

**Listen to your body—be safe—and
concentrate on your goals.**

SIDE NOTE: If you're new to working out, consider going to the gym at off-peak hours when it's less crowded. Low-traffic times vary wildly based on the gym you join and the community it serves, but going before the workweek rush (before 7 a.m.) or later at night (after 8 p.m.) is typically a safe bet. Ask at the front desk, and choose a time when you won't be distracted—or intimidated—by the regulars.

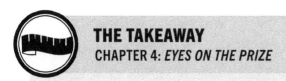

THE TAKEAWAY
CHAPTER 4: *EYES ON THE PRIZE*

This is your journey, not anyone else's. Don't waste time comparing yourself to others. Comparing your progress to someone else's is *pointless*. <u>You are you. You can't be anyone else.</u> Focus on bettering yourself.

The world wants to define your values for you. Don't fall for it. Stay mindful and present, especially when you look at photos in advertising and on social media. Everyone is selling *something*, even if you don't realize it.

People use social media to present a "best version" of themselves, which isn't always indicative of their truth. Social media platforms can foster jealousy and escapism. Don't rely on social media for motivation or inspiration. If you do, you risk measuring your progress against someone else's fake representation of themselves.

Don't compare your progress to others in the real world, either. Focus on *your* goals, not theirs. This isn't their journey. It's yours. Define your own objectives and then crush your goals by avoiding distraction.

You are your only competition.

CHAPTER 5

SO, YOU'RE NOT A KID ANYMORE?

It is a rough road that leads to the heights of greatness.

SENECA

DOES YOUR AGE IMPACT THIS PROCESS?

SHORT ANSWER:

No.

LONG ANSWER:

We live in a culture that covets youth above wisdom. That's a bummer, because getting older means you are alive, and being alive means you are lucky. *Getting older is a blessing. Period.*

It's true that your body is capable of different things at different stages of life, and that, in some ways, our bodies wear down as we age. You might not be as flexible as you were when you were 20. You probably don't produce as much testosterone as you did when you were 20, either. It will, most likely, be more difficult for you to gain muscle at age 40 than it was in your teens. But I'm not going to waste time telling you how your body might not perform "as well as" it did when you were younger. Why dwell on the past? There is nothing you can do about it now. Like Elsa says, "*Let it go, let it go.*"

Comparing yourself now to how you were when you were 20 is the same as comparing yourself to a stranger across the room. Both of those comparisons are futile. Everyone's body is different, and that includes the difference between your body at age 20 and your body today.

Your flexibility, strength, testosterone levels, metabolism, and so on are all primarily determined by your genetic profile. There is nothing you can do to change that. (Nothing safe or legal, anyway.) Your genes also determine how those factors change as you age. So why focus on how easy (or hard!) it was for you to [fill in the blank] when you were younger? Don't waste your time.

Your knees might not be as "greasy" as they were a few years ago. You might not be able to perform a deadlift because you were in a car accident last year. Or maybe you have even more significant physical challenges than that. Don't let those challenges stop you from making progress on your current goals. We all work within our limits in order to push those limits further.

Work at your pace in a way that targets the changes you want to see in the body you have today. If you suffer from back problems, avoid exercises that exacerbate the pain. But don't give up altogether just because something is busted or sore. If you can't run, walk. If you can't walk, try swimming. Never give up on being the best version of yourself that you can be today.

I guarantee you that, whatever your condition, there is someone out there who has accomplished goals similar to yours at your age. I know many guys in their 50s and 60s who just now achieved their ideal body type, and many of them came to fitness later in life. I also know people who endure physical setbacks that would sideline most of the rest of us, and yet they've pushed past these obstacles to achieve incredible goals.

It can be done. It can always be done. You only have to work at it.

You have control over one thing, and that is this:

You can control how hard you work at this very moment.

Your only job is to do the best you can do *right now*, today. Maybe it would have been easier to accomplish your goals when you were 20, but also it might not have been. Maybe you couldn't afford to join a gym when you were 20. Maybe you didn't have as much time because you had kids, or maybe you were in law school. Maybe someone in your family was battling cancer. Maybe you didn't want it badly enough because you were distracted by a dysfunctional relationship… *blah blah blah.*

Don't compare yourself to your past self. Don't live in the past. The past is gone. You are here now, and you must work with the tools you have at this moment. Your tools are different from the person sitting across the weight room from you, and they are also different tools than you had 20 years ago. Your tools are different from everyone else's, including your past self's.

Notice that I said "different" and not "better." Better is irrelevant. What you're working with right now is the best you've got. You at this moment are the best you've got, right now. *Use what you've got.*

Don't complain. Don't get frustrated. Show up and do the work.

I'm 40 years old, and I'm stronger than ever before. Today I bench press twice as much as I could bench when I was 20. I couldn't do a real pull-up until I was in my late 30s. My new goal is to make it to 10 consecutive pull-ups without assistance. I can do a handstand push-up now! If you'd asked me to do a handstand push-up when I was 20, I would have laughed or maybe cried.

You can't be the person you were 20 years ago, but you can transform the body you have today into the best it can be. I promise that is better than you've ever imagined it could be.

> *If you can't run, then walk. And if you can't walk, then crawl. Do what you have to do. Just keep moving forward and never, ever give up.*
>
> DEAN KARNAZES, *Ultramarathon Man: Confessions of an All-Night Runner*

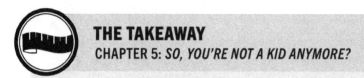

THE TAKEAWAY
CHAPTER 5: *SO, YOU'RE NOT A KID ANYMORE?*

You're lucky to be alive.

You're never too old to be the best version of yourself *right now*. Work with the tools you've got.

This is the only body you have. **Honor it.** Don't complain. Do the work.

Comparing how your body worked when you were younger is the same as comparing your body to a stranger across the room. Both of these comparisons are futile. *Let it go!*

There is always room for improvement, inside and out, no matter your present age.

That 20-year-old collegiate athlete on the bench next to you will be your age one day too. *If he's lucky.*

CHAPTER 6

OVERCOMING SETBACKS

Success consists of going from failure to failure without loss of enthusiasm.

UNKNOWN

I've been fighting a deadline at my day job, working nonstop for weeks. It's been almost a month since the last time I sat down to work on this book. I worked late on Saturday night, and when I got home, *I ate half a jar of peanut butter.* Then I spent Sunday alternating between eating handfuls of bacon, drinking bowls of granola, snacking on potato chips, and sleeping on the couch. I've been tired, cranky, and my willpower disappeared.

I experienced a fitness setback.

Even though I knew this month would be hectic, I intended to continue pursuing my goals. I purposely made a plan to eat well, and then I crumbled under the pressure of my stressful schedule. I heard the siren song of the peanut butter, and I let it draw me into the darkness.

Sometimes the closer you get to realizing your goals, the more obstacles the universe throws at you.

I wish I could say that I'm perfect and that staying in shape is easy for me once I decide to commit myself to a plan, but come on! We all know that's not the case for *anyone.* As much as it sucks, **setbacks are part of being human.** There are no ups without downs. Life is a roller coaster, not a slide. Work gets crazy sometimes. Stress happens. And then we eat foods that taste good even though we know they are poisonous—or, at least, detrimental to our health.

The thing to remember about a setback is that **you can always start again.** Right now is a great time. Here are three steps to getting back on track after you dig into the peanut butter jar at midnight:

STEP #1: REMEMBER THAT SETBACKS HAPPEN TO EVERYONE

Nobody is perfect. *Nobody.* So don't expect yourself to be perfect either.

I work a lot of freelance jobs. I'm grateful for the work, but it tends to overtake my life sometimes. My schedule is unpredictable, and I often find myself working seven days per week. Recently I accepted two new projects that I should have declined. I needed the money, so I agreed to take them on even though I knew I was acting out of fear (and greed).

In exchange for earning those dollars, I gave up most of my free time. The time I would have spent meal-prepping. The time I would have spent sleeping. The time I should have spent pursuing my fitness goals.

And then I got tired.

Yes, I managed to drag myself out of bed and get to the gym a few days each week. That was an achievement. But I also managed to overeat almost every day. **It's easy to overeat when you are tired.**

I gained five pounds this month. Ninety-nine percent of that is fat. It's hard to stay disciplined when it feels like I don't have the time to think about, let alone prepare, my food for the day. My goals flew out of the freakin' window.

Things like this happen to everybody. Life throws challenges at us. It might be your job or kids, or you might be dealing with depression.

**The first step to overcoming a setback
is to realize that SHIT HAPPENS.**

Sometimes you eat poorly, you stop exercising, and healthful habits disappear because you're stressed, busy, tired, or emotionally taxed. Sometimes setbacks are unavoidable...

Sometimes depression hits you after a breakup...

Sometimes you have a cold...

Sometimes you need to make money instead of exercising...

Sometimes your family comes to visit...

Sometimes you just slip.

Setbacks can last for days, weeks, or months. Maybe you've been in a setback for the past few years. Don't beat yourself up. Don't expect to be immune to the negative shit that interferes with life. You aren't immune. Nobody is.

STEP #2: KNOW THAT SETBACKS AREN'T PERMANENT

Don't wallow in a setback. A setback is part of the natural balance of the universe. Hard times will end, and it will get easier for you to achieve your goals. Setbacks aren't the end of the road. Instead, think of them as a wrong turn, and hear your inner GPS saying, "Recalculating" in that robot-voice.

Acknowledge that times are tough, and then get back to work as best you can.

Fight the temptation to abandon your goals. Quitting might seem more comfortable than accepting failure and then course-correcting, but what will feel better in the long term: giving up now or achieving your dreams later when things calm down?

Think about it this way: you need the lows to understand and appreciate the highs. Nothing is "good" without a point of comparison (i.e., something "bad" to compare it to). This idea seems convoluted, but it's simple. There is no "thin" without "fat."

How do you embrace that idea in practice? How do you use an abstract concept to get back on the horse and resume your fitness goals?

Acknowledge where you're at today, and then visualize where you'd like to be.

Start back at the beginning by visualizing your goals and putting together a new plan of action. You may already have done this last week, but it's time to do it again, *now*. That's the power and convenience of positive visualization: you can do it at any time, over and over again, and it becomes more powerful every time you do it.

Recognize the crappy way you've treated your body during this setback, and look at how those small choices have affected your larger goals. *Remove emotion from the equation.* You don't gain weight because you feel bad, just like you don't lose weight because you feel good. I know exactly what I need to do to achieve the kind of body I want. I understand the math, and I'm about to explain it all to you, too.

Setbacks happen, and then a window opens up—even a tiny crack—and you find the freedom and strength to start again. It might be challenging, but you always have the opportunity to start again. And again and again. **You have infinite do-overs.**

Don't live in a setback indefinitely. Don't fool yourself by thinking a setback is the new status quo. Just because you ate that bag of Reese's Cups last night doesn't mean you have to eat another one today. That brings me to the third thing you need to remember during a setback.

STEP #3: MAKE A NEW PLAN FOR MOVING FORWARD AGAIN AFTER YOUR SETBACK

I gained five pounds of fat this month. I'm not interested in making this extra five pounds of fat the new normal, so now I'm working on a *new* plan to burn it off.

I've acknowledged my setback, and I've chosen to recommit myself to my goals. Good news: I know exactly how to cut those five pounds, and I also know how awesome I will feel after I burn them off.

I choose to pursue that goal.

I choose to reclaim the energy those two jobs sucked out my life.

I choose to take more shirtless selfies.

I saw *Thor: Ragnarok* last night, and I choose to get jacked like Chris Hemsworth. I've made a plan to get there, and I'm excited to move past the setback I experienced this month. It's only a matter of time.

It's the same for you. Recommit yourself to your goals, renew your obsession, and then formulate a new plan. Base the math on where you are at today—post-setback—and get to work.

Your setback is just a setup for your comeback.

WILLIE JOLLEY

THE TAKEAWAY
CHAPTER 6: *OVERCOMING SETBACKS*

Setbacks happen to everyone. Life gets in the way. Life is hard. Don't beat yourself up when you fall off the wagon or when life makes it too difficult to stick to your plan.

Remember that **your setback isn't permanent**, even if it's lasted a long time. You can always get back in shape if you apply the rules in this book.

Don't wallow in your setback. Set new small goals. Then celebrate your small wins. Don't give up. Today is always a unique opportunity to try again. It doesn't matter what happened yesterday or the day before or the weeks before that.

Greatness can happen at this moment, right now. Your last setback is behind you. Now is a NEW opportunity to achieve a small goal.

PART TWO:

FOOD IS 90% OF YOUR PROBLEM

THERE IS ONLY ONE WAY TO LOSE FAT

*How long are you going to wait before you demand
the best for yourself and in no instance bypass the
discriminations of reason?*

EPICTETUS

CALORIC DEFICIT

Do you want to hear the secret way I transformed my body? Lucky you, I'm about to tell you how I did it. Here's the "secret" to fat loss:

To lose fat, you must maintain a <u>caloric deficit</u>.

A caloric deficit means you've burned more calories than you've consumed. That's the magic bullet! Later, I will walk you through how to calculate it, but here's a spoiler: the total number of calories you expend each day is called your total daily energy expenditure (TDEE). If you consume fewer calories than this total, you will be in a caloric deficit. (I explain TDEE in more detail later.) For now, just soak in the glorious truth that losing fat is simple and only requires one thing: *maintaining a caloric deficit.*

Why Is This Approach Special?

What makes this secret stand apart from all the other methods you've tried? The fact that it's not special at all. It's math. And it's 100% effective.

There are many people out there telling you what to eat and how to eat to lose fat. Some of them have good advice. Others peddle bullshit to sell you stuff. You might be reading this very book hoping to learn whose advice I listened to. I ditched 31 pounds of fat last year. *There must be somebody helping me, right?*

Nope.

Yes, I follow a plan, and yes, there are things I do to maintain muscle mass while losing fat. But here's the big picture: no matter the program, no matter the advice, there is only one way to lose fat. **You need to burn more energy than you consume.** That's it. It's physics.

Losing fat requires understanding a bit of elementary mathematics. There's nothing tricky about it. Energy "out" must be greater than energy "in." Any strategy for fat loss that doesn't explain how you create a caloric deficit is a gimmick. A ruse. A red herring. If a diet doesn't explain how it creates a caloric deficit, that's because it's creating one for you on the sly.

If a diet doesn't create a caloric deficit at all, then *the diet won't work.*

Some fad diets may retune the way your body processes calories by limiting certain foods or emphasizing others. These schemes might recalibrate your metabolism, but they still create a caloric deficit in some manner, possibly with dangerous consequences. The only ways to lose weight without being in a caloric deficit are to lose water weight (that's not fat, it's water) or to hack off a limb. Neither of those approaches is safe.

It's Physics

You can figure this out with Einstein's theory of relativity. *No joke.*

$$E = mc^2$$

The theory of relativity explains that energy and mass (matter) are different forms of the same thing.[16] They are interchangeable. The calories you consume are energy, and the fat and muscle you carry are mass. Under the right conditions, energy (calories) becomes mass (fat or muscle), and vice versa. Again, if you want to lose fat, energy "out" must be greater than energy "in."

- If you burn more calories than you consume, you end up with a deficit.

- If you consume more energy (calories) than you burn, you end up with a surplus.

- If the energy you burn equals the energy you consume, you maintain the status quo.

Calories that aren't utilized by your bodily functions are either stored (i.e., converted to fat), used to build muscle, or discarded via waste (i.e., pooped out). The reason you can't lose fat without being in a caloric deficit is the same reason you can't gain muscle without having some portion of calories you ingest directed toward building that muscle.[*]

There are nuances to how this equation works for each individual, but the sum always remains the same. To lose fat, you need to create a caloric deficit.

There Is No Secret to Losing Fat

You may be thinking, "Screw this! I came here for the special sauce. What does he eat, and what kind of exercises does he do?!"

Maybe you believe it's a waste of your time to think about the simple science I'm presenting here, but searching for more complicated answers sidetracked my fitness goals for 20 years. I bet you've already been down that road too. Talk about wasted time.

The plan I'm on now—the one that finally worked—got me the body I wanted *in three months*. It worked because I understood the math, and I committed myself to put this simple information to use every day.

There are apps to help you perform these calculations, but before you rely on an app, a trainer, or anyone else to tell you how many calories you should consume, you need to understand the underlying biochemistry. That way you can determine whether the advice you receive is valid or if it's total bullshit.

Stick with me. It's essential to grasp this uncomplicated science at its most basic level because losing fat is a lot easier than you've been making it out to be. Once you shift your perspective to seeing fat loss as calories in versus calories out, you can burn off that fat with minimal effort.

---

[*] Yes, it's possible to gain muscle while losing fat, especially if you are new to weight training. That's because your body is adapting to new stress. It's learning to redistribute the energy you might previously have stored as fat into new muscle tissue. It's possible, but only when you are starting out. It's an exception, not the rule. Don't worry about that right now, just focus on creating a caloric deficit.

QUANTITY BEATS QUALITY

It's not so much about what you eat; **it's about *how much* you eat.** The volume of calories you consume minus the calories you burn determines whether you are in a deficit or a surplus. This is a volume game. You cannot lose fat without being in a caloric deficit.

- Phrased another way: **you must maintain a caloric deficit to lose fat.**

There are countless studies of people losing fat on "diets" of fast food and Skittles. Remember the guy who lost weight while only eating at McDonald's?[17] (Does that sound fun to you? It makes me nauseous.) Sure, you will lose weight as long as you are in a deficit, and, yes, you can be in a caloric deficit while eating crappy foods. Is a McDonald's-only diet safer than Atkins? I honestly don't know! People wreck their system on diets like these all the time, but they still lose weight. How is that possible? Because *how much* you eat far outweighs *what* you eat.

Focusing on Quantity Is the Practical Approach

You can't always control the quality of the calories you consume. But you can control the *quantity!*

We live complicated lives. Sometimes your food options are limited. Sometimes your sister has a taco bar at her wedding. Sometimes your mom made a cake for your birthday. (Not my mom. She doesn't know where the kitchen is.) If you prioritize quantity over quality, you can maintain a caloric deficit without putting tons of restrictions on your diet. Sure, you want to make healthy choices… but do you know anyone who is capable of making healthy choices *all the time?* I don't! That's why creating a caloric deficit must be your primary objective.

More on Quality Later

Of course the quality of the food you consume impacts your body. You should eat foods that optimize your body's inherent mechanisms for energy expenditure. I cover how quality affects fat loss later in this part of the book, and I will provide you with guidelines for what to eat and when to eat it to maximize muscle growth (or prevent muscle loss) while losing fat.

However—one more time for the cheap seats—losing fat doesn't hinge on what you eat. Quantity upstages quality every time. If you eat fewer calories than you burn, you will lose weight—either fat or muscle or both—every time. *Always.*

There are two ways to ensure that the calories you expend are greater than the calories you consume. A hard way and a *right* way, as it were.

The HARD Way to Create a Caloric Deficit

When I say "burn more calories than you consume," I don't suggest that you create your entire caloric deficit by exercising. Many people attempt to lose fat with exercise, but that is the wrong approach.

There is a popular myth about achieving physical fitness that says you need to burn calories through exercise to lose weight. That is a misconception. Unfortunately, we've been taught to eat whatever we want—mindlessly, without purpose—and then to counteract the calories we consume with exercises. But get this: you don't need to exercise away excess calories if you don't consume them in the first place!

We don't need to exercise to burn calories.
Instead, we need to consume the right amount of
calories to support the activities we perform.

You don't need to run for hours or skip in circles around the parking lot of your CrossFit box to lose fat. While you *can* use cardiovascular exercise to increase your caloric deficit, you don't *need* to. Exercise is good and cardio has loads of other benefits, but relying on extreme amounts of cardio to inflate your caloric deficit is unnecessary, untenable, and boring as hell. *Who has the time for that?*

Plus, you can't always control how much time you have to exercise. Life gets busy. You probably have a job or a family. You have a limited amount of time to exercise each day (unless you are independently wealthy—lucky you). Don't predicate your caloric deficit on how much time you have to exercise.

Later on, I provide suggestions for exercising to build muscle, strengthen your heart and lungs, and increase your flexibility. For now, just know that **you do not need cardio to create a caloric deficit.**

The RIGHT Way to Create a Caloric Deficit

You can create a caloric deficit simply by monitoring how many calories you consume, and weighing them against the calories you burn. But how do you know how many calories you've consumed, or how they equate to caloric expenditure? There is only one way:

YOU NEED TO COUNT THE CALORIES YOU CONSUME.

That's it. That's how you lose fat. You need to estimate the number of calories that you consume, and you need to estimate the number of calories that you expend, and the latter needs to be higher than the former. Balance this equation by diligently tracking your calories, and you will lose the fat, regardless of how much you exercise.

That's the right way to create a caloric deficit.

You need to count your calories. *For real.* I'm repeating myself, and I'll repeat it again later: if you want to lose fat, you need to count the calories you consume. *All the time.* Not just when it's convenient or when you remember to do it. It's not hard. You don't need lab accuracy. You don't need to use a convoluted "points" system, either. You just need to track what you eat, how much of it you eat, and use that info to estimate the caloric value of everything you put in your body, to the best of your ability.

Monitoring the food you consume (i.e., counting calories) is 90% of the work you must do to lose fat. Yup, it's a little bit of work, but it's a hell of a lot easier than jogging for hours every day. It may sound tedious or time-consuming, but it becomes second nature to you very quickly if you are consistent and use tools that fit your lifestyle.

How to Count Calories

There are many new tools you can use to count your calories, both in and out. We used to rely on calorie books, but modern technology makes it much easier and faster than that. There are so many apps for tracking calories on your smartphone or computer. Do a Google search or check the App Store to find one that works for your lifestyle.

I use an app on my iPhone called MyFitnessPal. This app makes it very easy to count calories because it contains almost every single food you could imagine in its database—even restaurant foods.

If you're old school you can track with a notepad or fill out an Excel spreadsheet. Pick whatever works for you, and *be consistent.* It doesn't matter what works for anyone else. Choose a tool that fits into your daily routine and then make it a part of your life. For a while I used a custom form I created in Microsoft Word. I'd print out a bunch of copies and have it spiral bound at the local FedEx Office. Sometimes I prefer paper and pen.

Use the tool that makes it easy for *you* to track your caloric deficit, and stick with it.

> **SIDE NOTE:** In MyFitnessPal, it's easy to review your average daily caloric intake for the week or even the past month. Review that number instead of your calories from a single day when you fall off the wagon! Don't feel bad about consuming 5,000 calories yesterday or the Chocolove bar you polished off at 10 p.m. last night. Look at your averages from previous weeks to see how far off you have been on average. Now you have a more detached, objective view of the math.

Kitchen Scale

There is only one other tool I use for calorie counting, and that's a little digital food scale. It cost 12 dollars, and it resides permanently on my kitchen counter. I leave it out at all times, which makes it easy to weigh everything from nuts to chicken breasts without much thought or effort.

> **If you don't pay attention to how much your food weighs, you're probably overeating like the vast majority of people.**

Yes, weighing your food takes a little bit of time. But the accuracy you gain by weighing merits the few seconds you spend on this extra step. Once you've been weighing your food for a while, you'll be able to tell how much you've got by eyeballing it. For now, you need a food scale.

Own It

You might be embarrassed to use calorie counter apps and food scales in front of others. I understand that, but these tools help you reclaim your power over how much food you put in your body. Look at it this way: our current food industry is designed to obscure the quantity of food we eat. The more we eat, the more they profit. We're routinely duped into consuming way more calories than we need to consume. Using these tools helps you regain control over your body.

Don't be embarrassed by wanting to know how much you eat. Own it. If someone teases you for tracking calories or weighing food, take comfort in knowing that they are merely attempting to justify their ignorance.

Plan Your Calories, Too

Don't just use your calorie tracking tool to record calories; use it to *plan* your calories for the day in advance. This makes it easier for you to stay on track and deal with curveballs.

MyFitnessPal was on my phone for several years before I started using it to plan what I'd eat each day. I treated the app as a journal to record how much I hated myself—I mean, how much I'd eaten. I'd often overeat and then, sometimes, I'd enter that food into MyFitnessPal like a diary so that I could shame myself about what I'd eaten. I rarely looked at my total calories for the day, and I never even considered comparing my caloric intake week-over-week. I never made any changes to my eating habits, and I never adjusted my consumption. *And so my body never changed.*

Maybe you've been doing the same thing with your calorie tracker?

After several years of pretending to count calories in MyFitnessPal, I finally started to use it for real. I began meal planning, and I consistently tracked how much I ate every single day. That's when I finally started to lose fat. Most days, I plan my food for the day in the morning or the night before. If I'm on the road or have dinner plans, I look at the menu of the place I'm going beforehand. I decide what I plan to eat before I get there, and I adjust my other meals to balance against special events.

Don't get me wrong, I don't eat perfectly or "clean" all the time, but I find that the more prepared I am, the less likely I am to overeat. I like to obsess about the calories I consume, and being prepared for the unexpected helps to ensure my success.

THE TAKEAWAY
CHAPTER 7: *THERE IS ONLY ONE WAY TO LOSE FAT*

There is only one way to lose fat: **create a caloric deficit.**

Repeating this so it sinks in: **you must maintain a caloric deficit to lose fat.**

Quantity beats quality. What you eat is far less important than *how much* you eat. All matter is energy. *Where* the energy comes from doesn't negate this equation.

You need to understand how much energy you consume and how much energy you expend, so it's vital to **track the calories you consume every day** to balance this equation. (I'll show you the formula in an upcoming chapter.)

>   » Track calories in an app or a computer program, or write them down and add them up on paper.

>   » Do what works for your lifestyle, and be consistent.

>   » There are plenty of tools (e.g., apps like MyFitnessPal, calorie guides) that can help you gauge the caloric quantity of the foods you eat.

>   » I'd also recommend purchasing a small food scale and leaving it on your kitchen counter for easy access and use.

Do not rely on exercise to create a caloric deficit. Excessive exercise is unnecessary and untenable for most people—unless you are single, unemployed, or independently wealthy.

How much food you eat is 90% of this battle. Start with the calories, and everything else will fall into place.

CHAPTER 8

FIND YOUR STARTING POINT

You don't have to turn this into something. It doesn't have to upset you.

MARCUS AURELIUS

MEASURE YOUR BODY FAT PERCENTAGE

Before you can calculate your ideal daily caloric deficit, you will need an accurate measurement of your body fat percentage. This provides a benchmark for defining your goals, and is also critical to the formula I provide in an upcoming chapter. You can't devise a plan for losing fat if you don't know how much fat you want to lose. Fortunately, there are several options for measuring your body fat percentage.

You want the most accurate body fat percentage measurement that you can get, but not all of the following options will be available to all people. So, the most accurate measurement is *the one that is available to you.* Even if your number is inaccurate—and some measurements may be off by as much as 20%—you can still use that measurement to track your progress.

Determining your starting point is crucial. You can't know how to get where you're going if you don't know where you are at the start. Knowing your current body fat percentage determines your approach to creating a safe and effective caloric deficit.

Don't Be Scared

You might have a mental block against getting your body fat measured. It's embarrassing to have a stranger pinching your fat rolls in the middle of the gym, especially if that trainer is a super-fit model type. It's even more awkward to strip down to your underwear and sit in an egg-shaped plastic bubble while strangers watch you from outside the glass.

I can relate. I resisted measuring my body fat for decades because I was embarrassed. I avoided it even in the times I was seriously trying to lose weight because I was afraid of the truth. I was scared of that number. I was ashamed.

It wasn't until a few years ago that I finally faced my fears of body fat measurement and sincerely committed to the changes I decided to make. I was ready for change and I didn't want a little shame to get in the way of my success. I felt the fear and I did it anyway because I needed to see that number in order to figure out what I was doing wrong.

I did figure it out, and I transformed my life. *I'm not embarrassed anymore.*

Take the First Step

It can be hard to face the truth about where you are in this process. You're here because you want to change something you don't like about yourself, and nobody enjoys publicly acknowledging their shortcomings. But don't be scared of that number! Don't be afraid to admit that you've got work to do. **Be proud of taking this first step toward genuine, sustainable change.**

You are beginning your journey, and you need to know where you're starting to understand how to get to where you want to be. *This is true at any fitness level.* Even if you are healthy and trying to achieve "next level" fitness, you can't reach your goal without a baseline.

> You need to quantify and accept the things you
> want to change in order to change them.

The exciting thing is that this is your "before" moment. Consider how dynamic your "after" will be when you've accomplished your goals and can compare Future You to this Beginning You. *Can you imagine how proud you will feel then?*

Based on our discussions of the law of attraction, celebrating the small victories, and the "grass is always greener" principle, you know that the number one muscle you need to train to get fit is your brain. (The brain is not a muscle, I know. That's just an expression.) Train your brain to work through fear, shame, and embarrassment about your present shortcomings so that you can view fat loss from a logical, unemotional place.

There are many ways to measure body fat percentage. Here are a few.

THE DEXA SCAN

A DEXA scan provides the most accurate and accessible way to measure body fat for the average consumer. DEXA (or DXA) stands for Dual-Energy X-Ray Absorptiometry. Yes, it's an X-ray. That sounds intense, but here are the details:

- It uses about one-tenth of the radiation of a chest X-ray and .05% of the radiation in a CT scan.[18]

- That is comparable to the amount of radiation you are exposed to on a transcontinental flight. It's a meager amount of radiation.

- Despite the safety of these scans, pregnant women should avoid them to prevent exposing the fetus to any amount of radiation.

The DEXA scan was invented to test bone density,[19] mostly as a means of checking for osteoporosis without the need for a full-strength X-ray of the entire body. Fitness fanatics "saw the obvious value" of the DEXA scan as a general health and wellness tool, and commercial applications were recently introduced to the public. Now it seems like DEXA scanners are popping up everywhere, and the fitness community can't get enough of them. A machine that was only available in hospitals can now be found on a bus that will come to your gym to perform body composition tests in the parking lot! It's rad.

What's a DEXA Scan Like?

The first time I tried one of these it was on a bus parked near a gym on Sunset Boulevard. I stood in a dirty parking lot in my socks while I waited for my turn. Once I stepped into the bus, I was asked to lie face-up on a table and told to keep still for seven minutes. It was surprisingly easy and comfortable.

During the test, a giant wand passes slowly over your body, taking small, cross-sectional X-rays and sending that data to a connected computer. A few minutes after my scan I received the results along with a consultation to help me interpret them.

The information you get from a DEXA scan is incredible. I received six pages of very detailed data about my body composition. It included a visual outline of my body showing areas where excess fat had accumulated. It also revealed how much muscle I had—by the pound—in different parts of my body.

Holy shit, my left leg has 1.5 more pounds of muscle than my right leg! Time to hit the right quad a little harder.

You also learn about your bone density, which is important to know for general health. (Bone density increases with strength training, by the way.) Knowing bone density is especially helpful for women, because low bone density may be an early sign of osteoporosis.

I can't say enough positive things about this test. I've had seven DEXA scans in the past four years. Reviewing the results shows me the following progress:

- I went from 27% body fat to **10.8%** body fat.
- I went from carrying 48 pounds of fat to 17 pounds for a total loss of **31 pounds of fat.**
- I went from 123.4 pounds of lean mass to 134.9 pounds of lean mass for a total gain of **11.5 pounds of muscle.**
- My visceral fat mass dropped from 0.45 pounds to 0.13 pounds. (This might seem like a small change, but it's huge when we are talking about visceral fat, which is the dangerous fat surrounding organs.)

I was so proud to see these numbers because they proved that what I was doing was working.

How Much Does a DEXA Scan Cost?

DEXA scans used to cost hundreds of dollars, but the price of a scan has significantly dropped since they became available outside of hospitals. Visit

DexaScan.com and use the search function to see if there is a company that scans in your area.* They are popping up everywhere.

DEXA Scan Pros:

- An incredibly accurate and safe way to measure body fat
- Provides info about fat distribution
- Includes info about muscle mass and bone density in every area of your body
- Provides detailed analysis of visceral fat mass
- Multiple scans at the same location provide convenient progress reports for comparisons over time

DEXA Scan Cons:

- Radiation levels inadvisable for pregnant women
- Not available everywhere
- More expensive than calipers or a scale

FAT CALIPERS

You've seen these. They look like a pair of spring-loaded tongs. To use them, you pinch the skin on various parts of your body to measure body fat in different areas. In my experience, most trainers have a pair of these on hand because they are convenient and easy to use. The premise is that the thicker a skin fold is, the more fat you have in that area. You build a data set by sampling various body parts to create an estimate of your total body fat percentage.

As you can imagine, *fat calipers are not very precise*. Different people have different levels of elasticity in their skin—for instance, due to rapid weight loss, rapid weight gain, or the typical aging process—which causes an inher-

---

* I go to a place in Los Angeles called BodySpec (https://www.bodyspec.com). They currently charge $45 for a scan, and they give discounts for buying multiple scans in packages.

ent level of inaccuracy. You also need to be very consistent each time you measure, ensuring that you take measurements at the same locations, under the same conditions.

The person performing this test is, essentially, the machine doing the calculations. If you opt for this method, try to have the same professional measure you every time. This is the best way to ensure accuracy.

Fat calipers measure subcutaneous fat, but not visceral fat. Remember that visceral fat is the deep tissue fat surrounding your organs. It's the kind of fat that will kill you. You might be able to guess your visceral fat based on the amount of subcutaneous fat you carry, but again, this is a highly inaccurate means of calculating visceral fat. If your family has a history of heart disease, I recommend a body composition measurement that will give you a better picture of your overall health.

Still, if you are relatively healthy and only looking to lose those "last 10 to 20 pounds," fat calipers can provide a benchmark and are also useful for tracking progress. Plus, you can't beat the convenience or the price.

Fat Caliper Pros:

- Cheap and easy way to measure body fat
- Portable
- Readily available
- Provides a benchmark or a starting point

Fat Caliper Cons:

- Not very accurate
- Large margin for error between tests
- Doesn't measure visceral fat

BIOELECTRICAL IMPEDANCE ANALYSIS

With this technique, an electric current passes through the body to create a round-trip circuit. The speed of the current from point A to point B estimates the amount of fat in the body. This works because up to 60% of the human adult body is water.[20] Water conducts electricity easily, and most of the water in our body is stored in our muscles.[21] Meanwhile, fat is mostly nonconductive, meaning it slows the electrical current down. The more fat in the way, the slower the current moves.

Bioelectrical impedance analysis (BIA) gained popularity in the early 2000s, when it became easier to package the technology into consumer-friendly devices, like scales and hand grips. While BIA devices are more accurate than calipers in the hands of a non-professional, there is still a large margin for error—upwards of 10%.[22] The speed of the electrical current can be impacted by how much water you retain on a day-to-day basis. If you use a BIA device after you've been sitting in the sauna, there's a solid chance the test will be inaccurate.

BIA technology has indeed become more accurate in recent years, but the readily available consumer BIA products are mostly stuck in the past. The products like scales and hand grips only measure the current through a portion of your body. A scale you stand on measures "the flow of the current" through the lower half but only *estimates* fat content for your torso, while hand grips do the opposite. If you decide to purchase an at-home BIA product, look for one labeled DSM-BIA, or direct segmental multi-frequency bioimpedance analysis. These systems include separate lower and upper body measurements and are shown to have more accuracy than the older technology.[23]

As with calipers, any margin of error goes down with consistent, repeated measurements. There is always a benefit to repeating measurements, even inaccurate ones. Taking the average of several measurements will improve accuracy, and more data provides a more reliable benchmark.

Another downside to BIA testing is that it won't quantify different types of fat (i.e., visceral fat versus subcutaneous fat). However, BIA devices can't be beaten for convenience. I use a scale at home that incorporates bioelectrical impedance analysis. It's not a DSM-BIA, so it's much less accurate than a DEXA scan. (It consistently shows my body fat percentage to be *much lower* than that revealed by the DEXA scan.) However, I can still track changes every day, right from the comfort of my bedroom closet. By comparing one day's reading to the readings the scale has given me on other days, I can more accurately understand my progress than I would if I didn't measure myself at all.

You can't beat the convenience of stepping onto a scale when you get out of bed, and convenience fosters consistency. I weigh myself every morning at the same time (right after I brush my teeth). In theory, my body is in the same state of hydration when I wake up, so I take the measurement before I eat or drink anything. The scale connects to my WiFi network, so the measurements show up in the apps I use to track my weight, steps, and workouts. There is no simpler way to get a steady stream of data to track my progress over time. Again, *ease of use promotes consistency.*

BIA Pros:

- A fast and convenient way to measure body fat

- Easy to repeat consistently (daily)

- A relatively inexpensive initial investment

- Provides a number to start from, even though it's probably not the most accurate number

BIA Cons:

- Not as accurate as some other techniques

- Accuracy varies by manufacturer; older technology relies on estimates

- Doesn't quantify visceral fat

THE "BOD POD"

The Bod Pod[24] is a computerized device that looks like something out of *2001: A Space Odyssey*. According to the makers of the Bod Pod, it is an air displacement plethysmograph which uses whole-body densitometry to determine body composition (body fat and fat-free mass) in adults and children, and can accommodate a wide range of populations.[25]

You sit in a sealed, egg-shaped chamber (the "pod," duh) that compares the relationship among volume, pressure, and mass to determine your body composition. It can also measure thoracic gas volume.

The Bod Pod is a newer, more portable take on water displacement body composition tests. It's obviously easier to transport a person-sized, pressurized chamber than it is to transport a swimming pool. Its accessibility and portability have made it popular not only among fitness professionals but also in military applications.

I tried a Bod Pod at a CrossFit box three years ago when I was first starting my weight-loss process. I used the machine at the beginning of a one-month "food and fitness" challenge and then again at the end of the challenge. The results I received were an accurate comparison of my ratio of lean mass to fat mass. Like fat calipers and BIA machines, the Bod Pod tells you how much fat you have, but it can't ascertain how the fat is *distributed* in your body. You don't know how much visceral fat you hide, and it doesn't expose the ratio of *gynoid fat* (the fat around your lower body, hips, bum, and thighs) to *android fat* (the fat around your torso and upper body, like your neck, abdomen, and chest). At least with calipers you receive data from different points on your body (i.e., the various spots where you are pinched), and that data might provide clues to how your body distributes fat. My Bod Pod results included a single set of numbers—lean mass, fat mass, and estimated bone density—without insight into fat distribution.

The Bod Pod test I took cost me roughly the same as a DEXA scan. Despite its shortcomings and potential expense, the measurements provided by a Bod Pod test are very accurate. It doesn't give you the full picture, but it supplies a reliable starting point from which to track your progress.

Bod Pod Pros:

- An accurate way to measure body fat percentage
- Provides total ratio of lean mass to fat mass
- Less "invasive" than caliper testing
- No radiation

Bod Pod Cons:

- Can't pinpoint fat distribution or muscle mass by region
- Doesn't quantify visceral fat

FINAL THOUGHT

You have several options to choose from when trying to determine your current body composition. In many respects, you get what you pay for; more expensive tests, like a DEXA scan or the Bod Pod, yield more accurate results. With a DEXA scan you'll also receive more detailed information about where your body stores fat, and how much lean muscle you carry by region.

However, you can't bring a DEXA scanner or a Bod Pod home with you! Using repeated measurements to compile a bigger data sample makes it easier to determine if your fat-loss approach is working as expected. For this reason, I suggest combining an "at home" method for testing body fat, with semi-regular "laboratory" testing. (I say laboratory test, but DEXA scanners and Bod Pods are becoming more and more widely available in commercial settings that cater to fitness enthusiasts. They aren't just for labs anymore!)

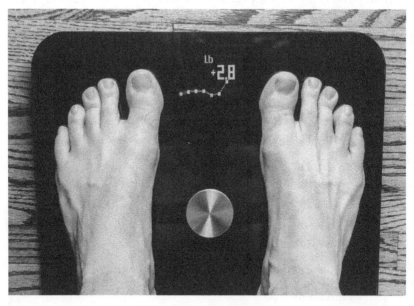

My morning check-in on a BIA scale.

THE TAKEAWAY
CHAPTER 8: *FIND YOUR STARTING POINT*

You need to know how much fat you have to lose before you start any fitness plan. You can't set realistic goals without knowing your starting point. For this reason, you should measure your body fat *first*, before attempting to calculate a caloric deficit.

I use a combination of twice-yearly **DEXA scans** and a daily **BIA scale** measurement to track my progress. This combo provides me with the accuracy (DEXA) and convenience (BIA) to build a reliable data set.

It's okay if a DEXA scan or a BIA scale is out of your reach. **Fat calipers** can provide a dependable baseline, and will continue to help you assess your progress over time, provided that the testing practice is consistent. Have a qualified professional perform the caliper test, and repeat the process with the same individual to ensure accuracy.

A **Bod Pod** is yet another extremely accurate test for measuring body composition. However, it won't provide you with details about *where* fat is distributed in your body. It also won't discover the amount of dangerous visceral fat you carry deep down.

I've benefited enormously by tracking my progress with these tools. Seeing the numbers change makes me proud of the work I've done. Invest in these tests regularly, and watch as the small changes you make every day add up to significant changes.

CHAPTER 9

CALORIC EXPENDITURE

Do what you can, with what you've got, where you are.

SQUIRE BILL WIDENER

TOTAL DAILY ENERGY EXPENDITURE (TDEE)

We need to consume a quantity of calories that supports the number of calories we expend, not vice versa. Calculating our consumption this way reminds us to **eat in order to support the things we do, instead of doing things to support the food we eat.** Life isn't about eating; it's about *doing.* Food fuels our activities, not the other way around.

For this reason, you begin your caloric deficit calculations based on how many calories you burn in a typical day. We call that your **total daily energy expenditure (TDEE).** Once you know your TDEE, you eat enough calories to support your activities while simultaneously creating a caloric deficit.

TDEE + Calories "In" = Net Calories

If you want to burn fat, your daily net calories need to be a negative number. *That's your caloric deficit.* For example, if my TDEE is 2,500 calories and I consume 1,900 calories in a day, that leaves me with a caloric deficit of 600 calories.

-2,500 (calories out) + 1,900 (calories in) = **-600 net calories**

To determine your TDEE you need—*that's right*—another equation. You estimate total daily energy expenditure by multiplying your basal metabolic rate (BMR*) by your average level of activity, which is represented by an "activity factor."

$$TDEE = BMR \text{ x Activity Factor}$$

So, what's your BMR and what the heck is an activity factor? I'm about to tell you.

BASAL METABOLIC RATE

Here's another "secret": you burn calories just by being alive. We each burn a default number of calories every day, regardless of what we do. We even burn calories while we sleep.

The default number of calories you burn every day is called your basal metabolic rate. Everything else you do during the day adds to the minimum number of calories you already burn by being alive. Any activities—from low-stress activities like sitting at your desk answering emails, to high-stress activities like kettlebell swings—add calories to your BMR based on your body's metabolic efficiency.

Knowing your BMR means you know the bare minimum number of calories your body will automatically burn every day, regardless of exercise. *It's vital to know your BMR to determine how much you need to eat every day.*

Calculating Your BMR

Your BMR is only an estimate, which means you merely need to figure it out to *the best of your ability*. All BMR calculations involve a little bit of speculation, and that's okay.

I believe the most accurate "at home" BMR equation is the **Katch-McArdle formula**. This formula factors in your current body composition, which is why I recommend that you test your body composition *before* calculating your BMR. (You read the previous chapter comparing body fat tests, right?)

Other formulas only account for height and weight, so they are less accurate because not all height/weight ratios are created equally. Muscle

---

* Also known as Resting Metabolic Rate (RMR). For our purposes, these terms are interchangeable.

tissue burns more calories at rest than fatty mass. Knowing your current body fat percentage aids in determining how much muscle tissue you have, and is therefore necessary to determine how many calories you burn as a baseline, without any activity.

The Katch-McArdle Formula:
BMR = 370 + (9.79759519 x LBM)

LBM represents your **lean body mass** in pounds. Your lean body mass includes muscle mass, bone mass, and basically everything that isn't fat. To determine LBM, you need another equation. *Oh good!*

LBM = Total Mass (in pounds) – Fat Mass (in pounds)

Determine your fat mass by multiplying your body fat percentage by your total mass. As an example, here's my calculation as of December 2014, when I was in the worst shape of my life. I weighed 177.5 pounds, with 27% body fat, so:

Fat Mass = .27 x 177.5 = **47.9 lb.**
Therefore, **LBM** = 177.5 – 47.9 = **129.6 lb.**

Plugging my LBM into the Katch-McArdle formula yielded the following BMR:

370 + (9.79759519 x 129.6) = **1,640 calories** (rounded up)

That number, 1,640, was integral to successfully calculating my caloric deficit. Once I knew it, I knew the minimum number of calories I burned every day, just by being alive.

However, it's dangerous to eat merely the bare minimum number of calories you need to survive. **Consuming calories equal to or just above your BMR is only advisable when extreme weight loss is necessary, under strict doctor supervision.** Most of us get off the couch and walk around and hopefully even exercise, which means we burn *more* calories than our BMR, so the baseline for calculating your deficit is based on your TDEE. Let's calculate that now.

ESTIMATE YOUR TDEE

Again, your total daily energy expenditure is only an *estimate* of how much energy you burn in a day. Don't sweat the accuracy because it's the best number we've got! As you continue on this adventure you will become better equipped to determine how big or small your deficit should be, based on the results of your experience.

As I mentioned a few pages ago, you estimate your TDEE by multiplying your BMR by an "activity factor." You choose your activity factor based on your typical activity levels. Assess your present, average level of daily activity, using the table below, and then multiply your BMR by that factor.

ACTIVITY FACTORS

1.200 = sedentary (You get very little or no exercise. You are a couch potato.)

1.375 = light activity (You do light exercise 1–3 days/week. You've been trying, but sometimes it's hard to get out of bed in the morning.)

1.550 = moderate activity (You get a moderate amount of exercise or team sports 3–5 days/week. You lift weights a few times a week and probably run on the treadmill on your off-days.)

1.725 = very active (You exercise hard, 6–7 days a week. You lift weights all week or hit that boot camp class every day. You're an animal.)

1.900 = extra active (You do arduous exercise *and* you also work on your feet. You are an Olympic sprinter, *and* you work in a concrete yard during the day. If this is true, then you're probably already jacked. Why are you reading this book?)

I recommend choosing an activity factor and then decreasing it by one level to start. *Step it back!* We tend to overestimate the calories we burn, especially during exercise. (Someone recently told me that their one-hour cardio class burns 1,000 calories. *I call bullshit.*) You don't want to cut calories too hard, but in my experience it's better to underestimate how active you are. That makes your deficit calculation a little less dependent on activity (i.e., exercise).

When I started counting my calories for real, I was going to the gym and running for 20 minutes, three days a week-*ish*. I might have been a "moderately active" person, but I calculated my deficit based on the "light activity" factor to start. Here's what I came up with:

TDEE = 1,648 calories (BMR) x 1.375 ("activity factor") = 2,266 calories

That number, my TDEE, was an estimate of the number of calories I burned every day, including time at my job and a little bit of exercise. Once I knew it, I knew that I was burning, on average, 2,266 calories each day.

Now that I've shown you the first variable in calculating a healthy caloric deficit, it's time to calculate how many calories you should consume to create a safe caloric deficit that will achieve your goals.

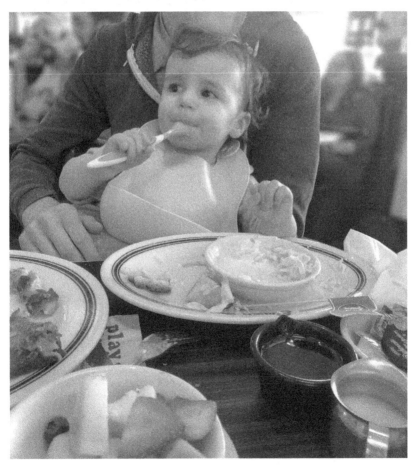

My son flexing his TDEE with a giant breakfast.

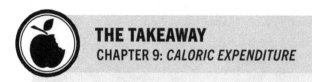

THE TAKEAWAY
CHAPTER 9: *CALORIC EXPENDITURE*

The total number of calories you burn each day is known as your **total daily energy expenditure** (TDEE). We will use this number to calculate a safe, healthy caloric deficit in the next chapter.

To estimate your TDEE, you need to know your **basal metabolic rate** (BMR). We use the **Katch-McArdle formula** to determine BMR based on your body composition.

» **BMR = 370 + (9.79759519 x LBM)**, where LBM stands for **lean body mass.**

» Your LBM is your total body mass minus fat mass. That's the amount you weigh minus the fat you carry. [**Total Mass – (% Body Fat x Total Mass)**]

You estimate your TDEE by multiplying your BMR by an "activity factor." This activity factor is a number that corresponds to your perceived level of daily activity; this includes the amount you exercise and how active you are at work, on average. *(These numbers appear a few pages back.)*

» **TDEE = BMR x Activity Factor**

» Since most people tend to overestimate their activity level, I suggest you choose a number that is one activity level lower than your self-assessment.

Once you determine your TDEE you can calculate your ideal caloric deficit. *(We'll do that in the next chapter.)*

CHAPTER 10

CALCULATING YOUR DEFICIT

*To bear trials with a calm mind robs misfortune of
its strength and burden.*

SENECA

Calculating your ideal daily caloric deficit requires balancing your fat-loss goals against your lifestyle, stress levels, and general state of mind. You need to create a deficit that you can achieve through small daily goals, and you also want to push yourself just the right amount so as not to give up. Speed vs. comfort. It's a trade-off. The lighter the deficit, the easier it is to adhere to, but the longer it will take for you to reach your ultimate goal.

I believe it's better to take it slowly—with a smaller deficit—than to give up on your goals altogether because you are exhausted and hungry. *Avoid the diet yo-yo!* Like I've already said, don't anticipate results. You will reach your target in time, no matter the size of your deficit, provided that you are consistent. Be patient and set smaller goals that you can *crush*.

Remember that this is not a "diet." Go slowly, methodically, and commit to incremental lifestyle changes every day. It's a new way to think about food. **Train your body to use food for fuel, and it will burn fat like a machine.**

I'm about to help you choose your ideal deficit, but first I should address the elephant in the room…

NO, YOU CAN'T STARVE YOURSELF

Maybe you're thinking, "I usually eat about 3,000 calories a day, so I'll fast for six days and then I'll be down at least five pounds. How's that for a caloric deficit?!"

Nope! It doesn't work like that. **You can't starve yourself.** Your body was designed to fight for survival. It is engineered to prevent you from losing fat that fast. That extra fat was intended to help you to survive for as long as you can without food in case you are stuck in the wilderness with nothing to eat. Or trapped on a boat without a fishing rod. Or the zombies have overrun the town, and you can't get to the grocery store, post office, evac chopper, etc.

Our bodies are inherently intelligent. Your body will vehemently resist any change to its current state of homeostasis, also known as its "set point." When you stop eating altogether, your body gets pissed off at you. Even if you lose weight, your body will wage a secret war to sabotage your efforts, and *eventually it will win.* It will do everything it can to convince you to start eating again.

And as soon as you start eating again, you will regain the weight you lost. In layman's terms:

Starving yourself makes it harder to lose fat.

Adaptive Thermogenesis

Adaptive thermogenesis is defined as a regulation of energy expenditure in response to a decrease in energy intake. It's another name for the way your body decreases your metabolic rate in times of lower caloric intake. That's right: your metabolism slows down when you don't eat enough food.

In order to protect itself from death, your body ceases to perform superfluous bodily functions and regulates your metabolism in favor of energy storage. You burn fewer calories overall and direct more calories to storage (i.e., fat) so that you have something to pull energy from when there is even less food around. **The less you eat, the harder it becomes to lose weight.**

There are still many conflicting opinions about the physiological impact of adaptive thermogenesis. Some research argues that the metabolic slowdown resulting from this process is a mere 5–10%. For some, that decrease is not significant enough to cause concern.

Other people take issue with the terms "starvation response" or "starvation mode" because they imply that your body slows down instantaneously—like flipping a switch—and that's inaccurate.

But those arguing against the idea of a starvation response or adaptive thermogenesis (or whatever you want to call it) miss the point entirely. Here are two opinions that provide a more appropriate definition of these terms and how they impact your fat-loss journey:

> *Starvation mode is a non-scientific umbrella term used to describe a cluster of scientifically-proven metabolic, hormonal, psychological and behavioral responses to extreme or prolonged calorie deprivation, which is common during many popular weight loss diets.*[26]

TOM VENUTO,

AUTHOR OF *Burn the Fat, Feed the Muscle*

> *The over 80% recidivism rate to pre-weight-loss levels of body fatness after otherwise successful weight loss is due to the coordinate actions of metabolic, behavioral, neuroendocrine, and autonomic responses designed to maintain body energy stores (fat) at a central nervous system-defined "ideal."*[27]

MICHAEL ROSENBAUM, M.D.

& RUDOLPH L. LEIBEL, M.D.,

COLUMBIA UNIVERSITY MEDICAL CENTER

There is much more to the starvation response than a disputed measurement of the *exact* percentage of metabolic slowdown that occurs when you starve yourself. The keywords in the two definitions above are "behavioral," "psychological," and "hormonal." In other words, there are mental and emotional ramifications to starving yourself. Starving yourself screws with your mind and your emotions, and that is why so many people ride the fat-loss roller coaster. **The starvation response causes the 80% recidivism rate many of us have experienced after otherwise successful efforts to lose weight rapidly.**

When you stop eating, your body says to itself, "Oh, shit! I better save my energy in case he doesn't find food! Wait, why is it taking him so long to find food? What is the friggin' problem? Oh look, there is food over there! I need it! I want it! Give it to me *now!*"

The last thing you want to do when trying to lose weight is to make it *harder* to lose weight. Duh. That's the problem with crash diets: you stop eating, you lose a few pounds—much of it water—and your body thinks something is wrong, so it halts your progress to protect you from starving to death. Your metabolism slows down, your hormones make you hungry, and your brain begins to obsess about food. (An unhealthy, subconsciously driven form of obsession, I might add.) You might get headaches, feel dizzy, or get nauseous. You will undoubtedly be tired.

As soon as you resume eating at normal levels, your body prioritizes fat storage for the next time it's starving. You stay hungry and your metabolism remains sluggish until you have convinced your body that there's plenty of food for the future. **You *overeat* in response to the starvation you've endured, and then the pounds come back.**

Additionally, research strongly indicates that this metabolic slowdown persists for a long while after periods of dynamic weight loss.[28] This is one reason why so many *Biggest Loser* contestants regain the fat they've lost so quickly after the competition.[29] Losing weight via extreme circumstances can be devastating for your body, both physiologically and psychologically. It wreaks havoc on hormone balance, metabolism, and morale.

In this book I mention the *starvation response* and *starvation mode* interchangeably to imply the whole picture of what happens when you starve yourself. Don't let anyone tell you that the starvation response isn't real. Scientists have documented and proven the yo-yo phenomenon for decades.

When you restrict calories past the point of starvation, your body will react appropriately to survive. What's more, your body doesn't differentiate between a very low-calorie diet and starvation. It will always push you toward maintaining the set point you've previously established.

The Cutoff Before Starvation

So, what establishes the "point of starvation"? How large can your deficit be before your body goes into starvation mode? Remember when I mentioned that your body uses a baseline amount of calories every 24 hours, regardless of your activity level? Again, this is called your basal metabolic rate (BMR), and you should consider that number as your threshold to starvation.

You never want your total caloric intake to be less than your BMR. If your BMR is 1,500 calories, you should never eat less than 1,500 calories in a day. If you do—regardless of how much fat you have to lose—you provoke a starvation response in your body.

**No matter your goal, you must always consume
a number of calories higher than your BMR.**

This becomes especially crucial when you try to lose that last 10 pounds of fat. The less fat you carry, the closer your body gets to freaking out when food is in short supply. If your internal cupboard is bare, your body will protect its reserve energy (i.e., stored fat) at all costs.

This Limit Includes Excessive Cardio Exercise!

Creating too large of a caloric deficit through cardio exercise is the same thing as starving your body by not eating. It's safe to employ a little bit of cardio to augment your deficit, **but you should never do so much cardio that your net caloric intake drops below your BMR.** If you do, you are starving yourself, slowing your metabolism, making your brain fuzzy, and inhibiting the functions that create muscle growth.

If you think running on the treadmill for two hours a day with moderate "dieting" is going to help you get in shape, you are wrong. Same for the elliptical, that Cardio Barre class, the TRX thing, and so on. You can starve yourself with extreme exercise too!

I've lost the bulk of my last 10 pounds with minimal cardiovascular exercise. On average, I do 10–20 minutes of high-intensity interval training (HIIT) three or four times a week, plus a few long walks with my family. (More on all of that later on.)

You don't need cardio to create a deficit, and you certainly shouldn't starve yourself by burning calories with excessive exercise. That's just another way to wreck your fat-loss plans.

CALORIES IN A POUND

Time for one more qualifier before we choose our deficit. To use this approach, you must accept that **there are approximately 3,500 calories in a pound of fat.***

While different foods have different nutritional composition, and though your body converts different materials into energy in different ways, a calorie is always a calorie. *Energy, baby!* Scientists have gauged that there are roughly between 3,400 and 3,700 calories in one pound of fat mass. Conventional wisdom assumes that you need to create a deficit of 3,500 calories to lose a pound of fat.

If you scour the Internet you will discover research to dispute that number. That's because fat loss is not a purely linear process. There are myriad factors that determine how each individual metabolizes food, and there is no one wholly accurate way to determine that specific number for everyone. The number of calories you need to cut to lose a pound of fat will vary based on how much fat you have to lose. According to Kevin D. Hall in the *International Journal of Obesity*:

> *[3,500 calories] approximately matches the predicted energy density of lost weight in obese subjects with an initial body fat above 30 kg but overestimates the cumulative energy deficit required per unit weight loss for people with lower initial body fat.*[30]

In other words, if you have a lower body fat percentage, your body probably requires a slightly larger caloric deficit to metabolize a pound of fat. If you are obese, you may not need a full 3,500-calorie deficit to lose a pound of fat.

But we don't need pinpoint accuracy to calculate a deficit that will work—3,500 calories is reliable enough. Why waste time nitpicking the accuracy of this number, when your caloric intake is merely an estimate, too?

You need to know how many calories to subtract in order to lose a certain number of pounds—3,500 calories per pound is an accurate estimate.

---

* That's 770 kilocalories in a kilogram of fat, for my friends using the metric system. For the sake of time, I'm going to present this in US customary units, but you can figure it out from there.

These calculations have worked for many people before you. You can always adjust your numbers later if you don't see the results you expect, but I doubt you are the exception.

CALCULATE YOUR DEFICIT

Finally, it's time to choose how much of a caloric deficit you will need to reach your goals. You need to decide how much fat you want to lose, how quickly you want to lose it, and balance those factors against how challenging you want the process to be. When you know how much fat you'd like to lose in pounds, you can divide the energy in those pounds across the time you'd like to be rid of them.

For example, if your goal is to burn 10 pounds of fat, you need to accumulate a caloric deficit of 35,000 calories (3,500 calories in a pound of fat x 10 pounds = 35,000). How you spread that 35,000 out over the course of weeks or months determines how quickly you will lose that fat, as well as how easily you will be able to hold on to (or gain) muscle.

- A higher daily caloric deficit means the fat comes off faster, but it will also be harder to sustain over time.
- A lower daily caloric deficit is easier to achieve each day, but it will take you longer to reach your final goal.

So what's the quickest, easiest, *best* way to lose fat? That depends on *you*!

Pick Your Priorities

First, define your end goal in explicit terms. You've already visualized how you'll look and feel when this is done, right? If you haven't, you need to. Set your ultimate goal, so that you can identify the small goals needed to get there.

- Do you have an important event coming up and you want to lose 10 pounds by that date?
- Do you have 200 pounds to lose, and you want to do it as efficiently as possible without crashing and gaining all the weight back?

- Do you want to look like 1970s Arnold Schwarzenegger, or maybe *Fight Club*–era Brad Pitt, and you don't care if it takes you the rest of your life?

- Do you want curves like Monica Bellucci or abs like Adriana Lima?

Specify for yourself *how much* fat you plan to lose and *when* you'd like to be rid of it. Define your ultimate goal as clearly as possible. Visualize how you will look and feel, and when you want that to happen. Be courageous but also realistic. Anything is possible, it just might take a little more time than you'd like.

How Hard Is Too Hard?

A person with 40% body fat and no experience strength training can get away with a more significant deficit than the person who is at 15% body fat. *Congratulations, newbies!*

However, most people struggle when they cut more than 30% of their TDEE. For instance, if your TDEE is 2,500 calories, a 30% deficit would be 750 calories, meaning that you'd consume 1,750 calories each day to create that 750-calorie deficit. A 30% deficit is difficult to maintain, and you will likely sabotage muscle. If you are already healthy and trying to lose the last 10 pounds (let's define "healthy" as less than 18% body fat for men and less than 22% body fat for women), I would not go above a 20% deficit.

But forget percentages for now. It's easiest for you to calculate your ideal caloric deficit based on your fat-loss goal in pounds, so here are a few example goals:

GOAL #1 – MAXIMUM FAT LOSS ASAP

If you have a lot to lose (>25% body fat for men or >32% body fat for ladies) and fat loss is your number one priority, you might aim to **lose two pounds per week.** Losing two pounds per week is the maximum I recommend, and it will be a struggle for most folks. *Nobody should ever try to lose more than two pounds per week.* More than that and you are most likely in starvation mode, losing water weight or muscle mass, even in cases of extreme obesity.

Based on our 3,500 cal/lb of fat estimate, two pounds of fat equals 7,000 calories, so if you want to lose two lb/week you need a **1,000-calorie**

daily caloric deficit. That's a big chunk of calories. In my case, implying a 1,000-calorie daily deficit results in this equation:

2,266 (TDEE) – 1,000 calories = **1,266 calories**

Uh-oh! Danger zone! CUE THE SIRENS!

That number, 1,266 calories, is well below my BMR of 1,648. (It's also a deficit of 44%, which is well above what I recommend.) Remember, if a **1,000 cal/day deficit** puts you under your BMR, that's too much, and it's unsustainable. *Don't even try it.*

Instead, here's what I suggest if a 1,000-calorie daily deficit (two pounds per week) pushes you past your BMR, but you want to shoot for the most intense approach possible. **Begin by trying to eat at—or just above—your BMR.** You already know that's the lowest you should go and, trust me, that will be tough enough.

In my case, it would mean consuming 1,648 calories a day, which would mean a 578-calorie daily deficit based on my TDEE.

Cutting 578 calories/day x 7 days = **4,046 total calories cut**
4,046 calories/3,500 calories = **1.15 pounds of fat loss per week**

For me, consuming calories roughly equal to my BMR yields approximately one pound of fat loss each week. If I've got an event coming up and I'd like to lose five pounds as quickly as possible, I know I should start *four to five weeks* ahead of time.

GOAL #2 – FROM "AVERAGE" TO FIT IN TIME FOR SUMMER

If you are already an average build (14–24% body fat for men or 21–31% body fat for women) and you have some experience in the gym, you might aim to lose one pound of fat per week as a comfortable target. That's 3,500 calories, which means a **500 cal/day deficit.**

For experienced folks, this approach will still challenge you, but it should be easier to maintain. It's what I'd recommend for those trying to reach their "next level" of fitness. It will be easier for those with a higher TDEE, and challenging *enough* for someone like me.

If you can manage to cut a pound of fat each week without losing muscle, you'll be down eight pounds of fat in two months. For an average male (165 pounds with 18% body fat) that takes you to 13.8% body fat in two months.

(29.7 lb of fat − 8 lb of fat) / 157 lb total mass = **13.8% body fat**

You *will* notice a difference in your body composition at 13.8%. In my experience, guys notice some abdominal definition around 12% body fat. But here's where it gets interesting…

Let's say you want to push yourself toward single-digit body fat in time to have a beach body. In the case of our average male above, if he gives himself a third month at this caloric deficit, he will be down to 11.5% body fat.

(29.7 lb of fat − 12 lb of fat) / 153 = **11.6 % body fat**

Twelve weeks to 11.5% body fat is not a lot of time, if you plan and maintain consistency. You can do this!

GOAL #3 – SINGLE-DIGIT BODY FAT THIS YEAR, BRO

Let's say you are already fit (<15% body fat for men or <21% body fat for women) and you are trying to get "ripped" (let's say anything less than 12% body fat) this year. You want to conserve as much muscle as possible, and you're willing to be patient. You might aim for half a pound of fat loss per week. It's an easier target, and you're less likely to catabolize muscle mass.

> **SIDE NOTE:** It's easy for your body to fall into starvation mode when you are already fairly lean. Don't starve yourself trying to get ripped. You can reach single-digit body fat with a goal of half a pound of fat loss per week, and you'll still have your muscle when you're done.

Half a pound of fat is 1,750 calories, or a deficit of 250 calories per day for a week. *Seriously, that's not a lot of calories.* It's totally doable. *Skip that effing Pumpkin Spice Latte and get over yourself. Do you want this or not, Cheryl?!*

As an example, a guy who weighs 170 pounds with 14% body fat will need to cut approximately eight pounds of fat to drop below 10% body fat:

(23.8 lb of fat − 8 lb fat) / 162 = **9.75% body fat**

Assuming he cuts 250 calories each day (all else equal) it will take him 16 weeks to reach single-digit body fat. If he wants to be even more conservative—maybe he's fighting to build muscle—he might slice that deficit in half to 125 calories per day, which would mean 32 weeks.

(125 cal x 7) x 32 weeks = 28,000 calories
28,000 / 3,500 = **8 lb fat**

Or, he could split the 250-calorie deficit (16 weeks) by taking an eight-week rest in between them. That would yield the same result (<10% body fat) in 24 weeks, while also providing eight weeks to focus on other goals.

The possibilities are endless. The point I'm making is this: if you break these giant fat-loss goals down into smaller, actionable goals, you can achieve *any* goal you'd like.

FINAL THOUGHT

Use your TDEE to set a baseline, then subtract the daily deficit you want to employ based on your goal and how long you want to take to achieve it. Use that ultimate goal to determine a comfortable daily caloric deficit (as long as that number isn't less than your BMR). Monitor your caloric intake diligently in MyFitnessPal or a similar tracker to make sure you stick to it, and prepare to be amazed as the fat comes off.

Once you decide on your approach, give it two weeks before you stress about how it's going. **A solid two weeks.** No cheating, no flubbing the numbers. Be as accurate as you possibly can be. If you don't experience the predicted fat loss (or close to it), something may be wrong with your calculation. Never fear, you know how to fix it based on the above. Consider your activity factor first. *Maybe you don't burn as many calories as you think you do.* Or perhaps consider increasing your target deficit, if you can maintain it safely and comfortably. There is a little bit of art to this and a little bit of experimentation because everyone's metabolism burns calories differently. However, **if you are consistent and track your caloric deficit, you will lose the fat.**

> **SIDE NOTE:** I suggest that you avoid "buying back" the calories you burn during exercise. There is no need to factor these calories into your deficit unless you are dangerously close to your BMR, or you are burning a large quantity of calories with excessive cardio. (You're not planning to do that, right?) It's tempting to add calories to your daily intake based on the number of calories that exercise equipment says you burned. Don't trust that shit! It will mess with your math.

Also, some calorie counting apps give you the option to increase your daily caloric goal after you exercise. If you use a fitness tracker in conjunction with a calorie counting app, I'd suggest you turn off the "exercise calories" function. Again, don't trust those machines to tell you how many calories you have left for the day. They default to overestimating TDEE, even when based on your heart rate, and they will likely sabotage your progress. Use apps to track your calories, but stick to your calculations for establishing your deficit. Above all else, listen to your body.

Be Patient

It takes time to reach your goals—maybe a few weeks or months, or maybe even a few years if you have a long way to go—but the time flies by when you aren't starving yourself!

Set small goals every day. Use those small goals to create your caloric deficit. Don't give up. Likewise, don't push yourself too hard. You've discovered a new way to think about how you eat, and it works if you let it.

I cannot believe what happened to my body in just three months of really monitoring my caloric intake. Three months was no time at all for me in comparison to 20-plus years of failed attempts and a constant yo-yo of fatness. And now I know exactly what do to burn the fat if my weight fluctuates again.

These results will last for the rest of your life if you want them to. If you're ready to make this change, just **follow the math!**

THE TAKEAWAY
CHAPTER 10: *CALCULATING YOUR DEFICIT*

NO, you can't starve yourself. A very low-calorie diet will provoke the starvation response:

» The "starvation response" is a catch-all term for a combination of **adaptive thermogenesis** (the slowing of your metabolic rate to reserve energy) as well as the behavioral, psychological, and hormonal ways in which your body adapts to starvation.

» The starvation response makes it harder for you to adhere to a fat-loss plan, and will likely lead to regaining the weight after otherwise successful weight loss.

Calculate your daily caloric deficit based on your fat-loss goal and how quickly you want to achieve it.

» **There are 3,500 calories in a pound of fat.** Multiply the number of pounds (of fat) you'd like to lose by 3,500. Then, divide that number by the number of days until you'd like to achieve this result. That number is your ideal daily caloric deficit.

» Push yourself just enough without sacrificing consistency.

» Don't try to lose more than two pounds per week, and never go lower than your BMR!

» Use small, daily goals to create that caloric deficit, and keep at it every day. Be consistent for at least two weeks before you assess how you're doing.

» If you aren't losing fat at the anticipated rate, adjust your activity factor or your target caloric deficit, and commit to that new plan for another two weeks.

Be patient. Rome wasn't built in a day.

CARBS & PROTEINS & FATS

Everything in its right place. In its right place. In its right place...

RADIOHEAD

Now that we've covered the single most critical factor in reaching your fitness goals—maintaining a caloric deficit—I can talk about the foods I suggest you eat and when I believe you should eat them. You know that by maintaining a caloric deficit you will lose weight. This is factual. But what balance of nutrients makes it *easier* to ensure the weight you lose is fat and not muscle?

Many popular diets suggest that by eliminating specific nutrients or food groups you can *trick* your body into burning fat. But these are mostly gimmicks. Remember that *what* you eat is always secondary to maintaining a caloric deficit. If you don't monitor your deficit every day, none of these suggestions will have a lasting impact on your goals. Some of these diets might even sabotage your health and well-being. If you want to control the amount of fat on your body, maintaining the deficit must always be your first objective.

Fitness professionals create fad diets so they can sell something unique. The keyword here is "sell." If I create an extreme diet that no one has ever heard of, I can brand it, market it, and sell it to all the sad folks out there who are desperate to try something they haven't tried before. (I was one of the people buying diets like that for many years.) Many also try to sell you special foods or supplements or tools that work in conjunction with the approach they have created. Again, the keyword is *sell*.

Your approach to choosing foods should incorporate the science behind how your body is engineered to use those foods. Let's consider the nutrients your body needs in greater detail so you can put together a "diet" that supports your lifestyle.

WHAT ARE MACRONUTRIENTS?

We define a macronutrient as **a type of nutrient the human body requires in large amounts.** Humans require three macronutrients, commonly referred to as *macros*. These are **carbohydrates, proteins**, and **fats**. Each macronutrient serves specific functions in your body, and these functions fall into two categories: *metabolic* and *structural*.

Metabolic functions provide (or exchange) *energy*. Energy exchange facilitates movement, big and small. The movement of your legs while you walk, the movement of oxygen through your circulatory system, and the movement of microscopic materials in and out of individual cells are all examples of metabolic energy exchange.

Structural functions are the functions of *matter*. If metabolic functions are movements, structural functions are the functions that build the things you move. This includes all of the cells that create your physical mass.

Your body requires both types of activity—metabolic and structural—to function. Your body is like a house; you can have all the cinder blocks in the world lying in a pile in the middle of the street, but you need someone to pick them up and assemble them in order to build the house. Likewise, a team of construction workers is useless if you don't have the cinder blocks they need for the project. You can't function properly without the supplies needed for energy *and* structure. These materials come from the calories you ingest.

As we've already covered, weight gain or loss relies on adjusting the balance of energy *in* to energy *out*. The calories you consume turn into one of four things during your body's natural processes:

- Energy to fuel movement, thought, and bodily functions;

- Matter that is used to build tissue, such as muscle;

- Matter that is stored for later energy expenditure (i.e., fat for another day); or

- Matter you expel from your body as waste (i.e., 💩).

All four of these processes are natural, and we require them to survive. Carbohydrates, proteins, and fats facilitate each of these four processes in distinct ways, in varying percentages that differ for each person's body.

Did you fall asleep yet? I hope not. I know this seems tedious, or like a throwback to junior high health class, but it's important knowledge that will inform your food choices. How can you decide to "cut carbs" or "carbo-load" without knowing how that decision will affect your bodily functions? Understanding how and why you balance your macronutrients allows you to make mindful food choices. Each one serves a purpose, and you should know its purpose before you adjust how much you consume.

CARBOHYDRATES

A carbohydrate is a molecule with a 2:1 ratio of hydrogen to oxygen, similar to water (H_2O). "Carbohydrate" is also a synonym for "saccharide." The carbohydrate class of molecules includes sugars, starches, and cellulose. These range from simple sugars (monosaccharides) to more complex starches and glycogen (polysaccharides).

Polysaccharides take longer to break down. They are digested slowly for sustained energy over longer periods of time, or stored as fat that can be converted into energy later as needed.

Simple carbohydrates metabolize quickly. They break down fast, meaning the body converts them into energy right away. However, any excess calories not converted to energy can and will be stored for later use through fat conversion. This includes simple carbohydrates that aren't utilized rapidly after consumption.

Cellulose is the primary material used to build cellular walls. In food terms it's commonly referred to as "fiber." Cellulose is an insoluble substance. We can't digest it, but ingesting it helps us to move waste through our bodies, including excess fat. Vegetables contain lots of cellulose, as do whole grains, and these foods maintain digestive regularity. They also promote healthy cholesterol levels and a proper triglyceride balance in the bloodstream. (Heart disease is still a leading cause of death, and consuming fibrous carbohydrates can go a long way to prevent it.)

In dietary terms, when people refer to "carbohydrates" or "carbs" as a food source, they are talking about the food group most commonly associated with this macronutrient. Foods known as carbs are those containing a high concentration of carbohydrate molecules.

Carbohydrates and Energy (ATP)

Carbohydrates are like the construction workers in our house-building analogy. We primarily need carbohydrates for metabolic (energy related) functions. Carbs are essential. *Here's a little science. Skip ahead if you're bored.*

ATP (adenosine triphosphate) is the molecule our bodies use at the intracellular level to shuttle energy between cells.[31] ATP molecules contain a chain of phosphates. These molecules release energy (in the form of heat) when the bonds between the phosphates are broken via hydrolysis. All cellular functions require ATP. That includes, ultimately, all of your bodily functions. ATP is necessary for everything you do—from breathing to moving your eyes to, of course, lifting weights. **ATP creates the energy you need to live.**

Carbohydrates yield the bulk of the ATP we need, through the digestion/oxidation process. Glucose, in particular, is the primary source of ATP in animal life.[32] While the body can derive ATP from fat and, to a much lesser extent, protein, **carbohydrates are the most efficient source of cellular energy.**

Carbs Get a Bad Rap

So why do carbs have a bad reputation among some dieters? Carbohydrates have gotten a bad rap in the past decade or so because Western society eats the wrong kinds of carbs at the wrong time, which leads to weight gain and metabolic disorder. We often tend to eat sugary foods at times of low energy expenditure, causing unnecessary blood sugar spikes and encouraging the body to store those sugars as fat.

However, carbohydrates aren't *evil*, as some folks make them out to be. On the contrary, your body was designed to utilize carbs, so don't throw the baby out with the bathwater—as many low-carb diets do. You need to consume carbohydrates when your activities merit it, instead of giving up on them altogether.

The Insulin Response

Insulin is a hormone created by the pancreas. It regulates blood glucose (sugar) levels by prompting cells in your body to pull excess glucose from your bloodstream. This includes muscle, which is why the insulin response (i.e., your body's mechanism for releasing insulin) is super important for building muscle. Muscle fibers include insulin receptors. Insulin molecules attach to a muscle cell, allowing the muscle to absorb glucose and amino acids, which triggers protein synthesis and muscle repair.

Without insulin, your muscles wouldn't increase in size. It's important to consider the impact of carbohydrates—especially simple carbohydrates—on the insulin response system and, therefore, strength-training goals. In layman's terms: *carbohydrates are essential for muscle growth!*

Insulin Resistance

Here's the dark side of the insulin response system. Diets high in simple sugars can overload the body's ability to regulate blood sugar, leading to *insulin resistance*. Insulin resistance occurs when cells do not respond well to insulin—meaning higher levels of glucose remain in the bloodstream—and it is a precursor to diabetes.[33] It's best to avoid diets high in simple carbohydrates that aren't consumed in conjunction with higher activity levels. For this reason I limit simple carb consumption to periods of high energy expenditure (i.e., when I exercise).

Conversely, diets high in complex carbohydrates (oats, etc.) and fibrous carbohydrates (leafy green vegetables) have been shown to decrease the risk of diabetes.[34] Leafy green vegetables are safe to consume at any time during the day.

Carbs and Gut Bacteria

The current popularity of low-carb/ketogenic diets has stirred up further study of the impact of carbohydrates on gut bacteria. Some studies have found that ketogenic diets lowered the diversity of gut bacteria and led to an "increased amount of pro-inflammatory bacteria."[35] One study showed that a fat-exclusive diet "led to a substantial decrease in the production of short chain fatty acids and antioxidants in the colon," which could have negative health consequences.[36] There are potentially positive effects to a ketogenic diet in cases of insulin resistance or extreme obesity, however it appears that the effects of a low-carb diet on gut bacteria should give you pause before deciding to eliminate carbohydrates from your diet completely.

Glycemic Index vs. Glycemic Load

You may already be familiar with the glycemic index (GI). It's a scale from 0–100 that ranks the effect of a food on your blood sugar level, where 100 represents pure glucose. The scale has been used by diabetics for decades in order to anticipate the need to supplement insulin after eating certain foods. The problem with the GI is that it doesn't take into account the amount of carbohydrate included in a *serving* of the food, which may also include water, fiber, etc.

Enter the **glycemic load** (GL) scale. This scale factors in the composition of a food by dividing the GI by 100 to create a percentage, then multiplying that by the total number of carbohydrates (minus the fiber) in a serving of that food. It's a much more sensible way to gauge the effect of foods on your blood sugar. The grocery shopping list I've included at the back of this book lists carbohydrate foods in order of GL. This, in combination with your food tracking app, provides a better idea of how to time carbohydrate intake based on activity levels.

Carbohydrate Pros:

- Carbs are your body's primary source of energy.
- Simple carbs, a.k.a. high-GL carbs, supply the energy needed for exercise and also facilitate the insulin response required to transport other essential nutrients to muscles.
- Fibrous carbohydrates aid in digestion and help move excess fat and cholesterol out of the body.

Carbohydrate Cons:

- When timed incorrectly, carbohydrates can be stored as fat.
- An excess of high-GL carbohydrates in your diet can cause insulin resistance, leading to diabetes and other health concerns.

PROTEINS

Like carbohydrates, protein molecules come in different variations that serve different bodily functions.

Some proteins are enzymes. Enzymes catalyze (or "fire up") biochemical reactions during the metabolic process, which helps us to break down other molecules. As an example, lactase is the enzyme that breaks down lactose, the sugar found in milk. Without lactase we cannot turn lactose into energy.

Beyond enzymes, though, most proteins have structural or mechanical functions used to build our tissue at the cellular level, starting with the cytoskeleton that gives a cell its shape. In our house analogy, you should think of proteins primarily as the cinder blocks you need to build your body.

We Need Protein

Proteins are chains of amino acids. Nine different amino acids are essential for your body to function. You need those cinder blocks in your body so the construction workers have material to build your house. (Who else is tired of the house-building analogy?)

Nine Essential Amino Acids

Histidine: enables growth, the formation of blood cells, and tissue repair

Isoleucine: regulates blood sugar; helps with wound healing, immunity, and hormone production

Leucine: repairs muscle tissue, regulates blood sugar

Lysine: builds muscle; regulates hormones, antibodies, and enzymes; produces elastin and collagen

Methionine: strengthens skin and hair; helps absorb zinc and selenium

Phenylalanine: converted to tyrosine, dopamine, epinephrine, and nor-epinephrine; used in brain functions

Threonine: used in collagen, tooth enamel, and skin elastin; helps metabolize fat, boost immunity

Tryptophan: a precursor of serotonin (sleep) and melatonin (skin pigmentation/sleep)

Valine: essential for the central nervous system: cognition, coordination

The above amino acids are commonly referred to as "essential" not only because your body requires them, but also because you must *ingest* them. Humans cannot biosynthesize these nine essential amino acids, so our bodies rely on food to supply them.

In dietary terms, when people refer to "proteins" as a food source, they mean the food group most commonly associated with this macronutrient (i.e., foods that have a high concentration of proteins). Animal sources are the most common form of protein we can eat. They are the easiest, most readily accessible sources of these amino acids.

Don't hate me yet, vegetarians. Yes, I'm an omnivore, but I've been vegetarian, and I was a pescatarian (vegetarian with the exception of fish) for 12 years. I currently prefer an omnivorous diet for the sake of convenience. However, you can derive all nine essential amino acids from a vegetarian diet. There are four "hard to find" amino acids that are missing from most plant foods. These are lysine, tryptophan, methionine, and phenylalanine. Vegetarians can find them in quinoa, soy products, chia seeds, etc. The challenge for vegetarians is ensuring they consume *enough* of these amino acids, and that is beyond the scope of what I'm willing to write about here. If you're vegetarian, you need to make sure you eat a variety of foods that cover all of the amino acids you need. Look 'em up and incorporate the data into your food planning.

Too Much Protein

High-protein diets may prompt several health risks. In particular, weight gain and higher total death risk are significantly associated with diets that replace carbohydrates with dietary protein.[37] These risks likely rise as a result of increased saturated fat found in animal products, but excess protein is also typically stored as fat. There are also studies linking diets high in red meat to increased cancer risk,[38] kidney damage in individuals with preexisting kidney disease,[39] and kidney stones.[40] High-protein diets where protein intake replaced fat intake do not yield the same level of risk.

Protein Pros:

- Protein is essential for every cell in your body.

Protein Cons:

- Protein is not an efficient source of energy.

- High-protein diets are linked to several health risks, although these concerns may be exacerbated by diets with greater consumption of red meat and foods which are high in saturated fat.

FATS

Fats (i.e., *triglycerides*, a type of lipid) serve both metabolic and structural functions in the body. Triglycerides can be converted into energy quickly, but they can also be stored for later use.

The fat you are trying to lose is there because your body decided to store triglycerides. Your body creates these "storage units" of triglycerides from excess food. That's what fat is. Think of the excess fat you're carrying as something your body thought of as a *backup*. It's not your enemy, and it's not an accident. *It's there because your body thought you'd need it later.* Why else would you have eaten that entire pizza unless you were saving up for winter hibernation, right?

In terms of your diet, when people refer to "fats," they mean the food group composed primarily of this macronutrient (i.e., foods that have a high concentration of fats).

We Need Fat

You might ask yourself, "Self, if my body can synthesize fat, do I still need to eat it?" *Yes, you do need to ingest fats.* In particular, two types of essential fatty acids are not synthesized by the human body: omega-3 and omega-6 fatty acids. Again, these are called *essential* because you need them in your body and because they can't get there if you don't ingest them.

Omega-3 fatty acids are used by your brain, skin, and eyes; to fight inflammation; and more. They also reduce the number of *other* triglycerides from your bloodstream. These are fats that keep you thin! Some omega-3 fatty acids include α-linolenic acid (found predominantly in nuts and plants) and both eicosapentaenoic acid and docosahexaenoic acid, which show up in fish and other sea creatures. Typically, our primary dietary source of omega-3 fatty acids is fish.

Omega-6 fatty acids enable cellular repair and production and limit inflammation in the healing process. Weight training is a process of damaging and repairing muscle tissue to promote growth, so it stands to reason that omega-6 fatty acids are a valuable part of the muscle-building process. Omega-6 fatty acids show up in poultry, eggs, and (to lesser degrees) in nuts, seeds, and some plant matter.

In addition to supplying these essential fatty acids, dietary fats provide energy over extended periods because they take longer to digest than carbohydrates. Fats are dense, which helps you to feel *full* longer, while also supplying a steady flow of energy without provoking the insulin response.

The Types of Fat

Instead of trying to explain the molecular differences between various forms of fats, I'll give you the two primary kinds of dietary fat and how they appear in foods we eat:

Saturated fat: Think of this as *thick* fat. It's like the fat you have to cut off a New York strip steak. Saturated fat molecules have a high melting point and thus are typically solid at room temperature. They take shape and hold it. Saturated fats include most animal fats, as well as some vegetable fats like coconut oil.

Unsaturated fat: Think of this as oil, or the oils in foods like nuts and seeds. These molecules have at least one double bond, which creates a lower melting point. Since the melting point is lower, unsaturated fats are not solid at room temp; they melt into oil. Unsaturated fats can be monounsaturated (meaning they have one double bond) or polyunsaturated (several double bonds). Examples of foods that are high in unsaturated fats include most nuts, fish, and cooking oils that originate from plants.

You probably just gleaned that omega-3 and omega-6 fatty acids are unsaturated fats. You are correct! These fats have a lower melting point than saturated fats, and they are the healthiest type of fat you can eat. When you plan your macronutrient intake, **remember to favor unsaturated fats over saturated ones**. A small amount of saturated fat in your diet is fine, but diets high in saturated fat are associated with heart disease, diabetes, cancer, and other adverse conditions.

Limit Extra Fats Found in Packaged Foods

You've no doubt heard health nuts talking about how they avoid packaged foods (i.e., foods that come already prepared, in a wrapper). But *why*? What's wrong with a little convenience?

Here's why packaged foods are problematic: when companies manufacture packaged foods, they prioritize transportation, longevity, and their bottom line. They create food products that are designed first and foremost for the industrial food supply chain, *not necessarily for the human body*. How does this process affect those foods? **Packaged foods are often high in saturated fats.** Saturated fats have a higher melting point, so they hold up better during transportation. The saturated fats in packaged food retain their shape and consistency while traveling across the country in a semi truck on a hot day. If these items contained mostly unsaturated fats, they would likely fall apart as the fats melted during transport.

Packaged dessert foods (cookies, pies, Twinkies, and so on), baked goods, and maybe even your favorite protein bar are made with saturated fats so that they survive the turbulent trip from the factory floor to grocery store shelf. Sometimes the saturated fat content increases well beyond what's necessary, only to ensure product stability. *Gross.*

There are many other reasons to avoid prepackaged foods as much as possible, but high saturated fat is a primary cause for concern. If the thing you are about to eat has a label, *always read it*. Avoid unnecessary saturated fat at all costs. Not only is it bad for you, but it will quickly sabotage your caloric deficit.

I've included a list of recommended fats at the end of the book. Choose wisely and you will make your body happy as it learns to cut your own saturated fat from your waistline.

Fat Pros:

- Stored fats provide energy during exercise (after simple carbohydrates are metabolized).

- Fats aid in vitamin absorption.

- Fats help you feel "full," so you don't overeat.

- Certain mono- and polyunsaturated fats reduce your levels of bad cholesterol (LDL), which helps to prevent heart disease.

Fat Cons:

- Fats are the most calorically dense macronutrient, meaning there are more calories per gram. (I'll define this more clearly in the next chapter.)

- Excess saturated fats and trans fats lead to higher levels of LDL cholesterol in the system, which often results in heart disease.

- Diets high in saturated fats are linked to diabetes, cancer, and other serious health risks.

FINAL THOUGHT

Your body is designed to use all three of these macronutrient groups for different reasons, at different times. Do not be tempted by diets that eliminate one of these macronutrients as a means to fat loss.

To lose fat efficiently and keep it off, you need to create the right balance of all three macronutrient groups, based on your activities, lifestyle, and fat-loss goals. Cutting out a macronutrient group is not a substitute for a caloric deficit.

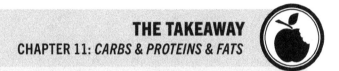

THE TAKEAWAY
CHAPTER 11: *CARBS & PROTEINS & FATS*

There are three macronutrient groups in the human diet: **carbohydrates**, **proteins**, and **fats**. All three macronutrient groups serve specific functions in your body, and all three are essential.

» **Carbohydrates create energy**, both quickly and over extended periods of time. Carbohydrates also provoke the insulin response, which regulates glucose in the bloodstream, facilitates protein synthesis for muscle building, and stores excess nutrients for later use.

» **Proteins are the building blocks of your body.** We require them for all tissue growth and repair, including muscle tissue.

» **Fats work in multiple ways.** They can provide energy over longer periods, and fatty acids support brain function, cellular repair and reproduction, and also reduce inflammation.

Consume each macronutrient in proportion to your current activities. Doing so allows your body to maximize each one for its intended functions, and limits the chance that excess nutrients are stored as fat.

FINDING THE RIGHT MACRONUTRIENT BALANCE

To put everything in balance is good, to put everything in harmony is better.

VICTOR HUGO

I covered the three macronutrient groups in the last chapter—proteins, carbohydrates, and fats. If you read that chapter you know that each of these macronutrients is essential to the human body. Your body works best on a diet that includes each of these three macronutrient groups. It's designed to work that way. Any diet that excludes one of these groups in totality will shortchange your body's natural processes.

Let's cover how much of each macronutrient you should consume for optimal fat loss. The way to determine this is to explore and understand the concept of *caloric density*.

Caloric density is the ratio of calories to mass.

The caloric density of food—or, in this case, a macronutrient—is the ratio of calories to the mass of the food. Foods with high caloric density have more calories per mass, and foods that are less calorically dense have fewer calories.

Calorically speaking, macronutrients are not created equal. Each of these macronutrients has a different caloric density that contributes to your total caloric intake every day. Here are the caloric values of each macronutrient as commonly accepted:

1 gram of protein = 4 calories
1 gram of carbohydrate = 4 calories
1 gram of fat = 9 calories

What information can we glean from these three significant numbers—4, 4, and 9? We see that proteins and carbohydrates are *less* calorically dense than fats. You can eat more than twice as many grams of protein or carbohydrate in exchange for the same amount of calories of fat. In other words, there are 2.25 times as many calories in one gram of fat than there are in one gram of protein or carbohydrate.

Yes, fats are more calorically dense, but they are also more physically dense. That means they have more mass and will, therefore, make you feel fuller *faster*. A little bit of fat goes a long way toward meeting your caloric needs and making you feel full.

Of course, **these numbers apply to macronutrients in their purest form.** But when was the last time you had a fat-free steak? How about a doughnut that wasn't fried in fat? It's not easy to classify any single food item as a fat, a carb, or a protein. The foods we eat and the recipes we prepare use a combination of these macronutrients. That's why it's imperative to record the macronutrient breakdown of the prepared foods we eat, not just the food group we casually associate them with.

TIMING YOUR MACROS

How much of each macro you need each day depends on your activity level and how the body uses each of these nutrients for the activities you perform. If each macronutrient serves specific functions, it stands to reason that you should consume them at times when those functions are happening in your body.

Here are a few thoughts on when to prioritize each macronutrient, based on your daily activities. For the sake of argument, let's assume that we can consume each macronutrient in its purest form.

Carbohydrates

Carbohydrates metabolize rapidly, so it's best to consume them when you need energy.

High-GL carbs are best utilized during or immediately after exercise. This approach applies to both cardiovascular exercise and strength training. That's the time when your body needs to replenish the glycogen stores in its muscles because it's been using that glycogen to exercise. It's also the best time to stimulate an insulin response so that your body can shuttle protein to the muscles you've just worked. Simple carbohydrates include natural options such as fruit, maple syrup, and table sugar, as well as processed options like sports drinks, carbohydrate powders, candy, and anything with added sugar.

Complex carbs should be consumed throughout the day when you're awake but not necessarily exercising. You digest complex carbs more slowly than simple carbs, but they provide your body with the long-term energy it needs to move, work, and think during times of less activity. Complex carbohydrates include foods like vegetables, legumes, and whole grains like brown rice, oats, and barley. (I don't consider refined grains to be complex, and I explain my reasons for that in a subsequent chapter.)

Protein

Lean protein can be consumed at any time during the day and is typically a safe go-to, provided that the accompanying fat content is low. Some people swear they experience more notable muscle gains when they incorporate a quick-digesting protein, like whey protein powder, immediately following their workouts. That's part of my current routine. However, the scientific merits of this timing are debatable. Some studies indicate that you can consume protein at any time of day with the same great results. The important thing is to ensure that you consume enough protein throughout a 24-hour period.

Fat

Fats are filling because they are calorically dense. That means you can eat less of them and be satiated. For me, the optimal time to consume fats is later in the day—before bed, for instance—when I will consume fewer calories overall but I would also like to feel full.

When to Limit (or Avoid) Each Macro

I told you that the quantity of calories you consume is more important than the *quality* of calories. But that doesn't mean *what* you eat doesn't contribute to your fat-loss goals. It does. In particular, people gain fat by consuming foods at the wrong time. This is especially true of excess simple carbs, which we know are easily stored as fat. You should limit high-GL carbs in times when your body won't use them, such as when you are resting.

Eating simple carbs late at night is a chief contributor to the overfat epidemic. We've all been trained to eat sweets and high-glycemic snacks right before bed, often while we sit stationary in front of the television. Guess what? *Eating potato chips and ice cream before bed will make you fat.* Eating carbs when we aren't moving trains our body to store those carbs as fat.

On the other hand, we know that protein doesn't easily convert into energy, and it takes longer to digest. You should prioritize overall protein intake for muscle building, but you *don't* need to consume protein before a workout. Protein doesn't provide the energy you need to exercise. You need carbohydrates when training. *Those might even be high-GL carbs.*

Similarly, you need *complex* carbs for sustained energy and focus during work hours. Protein is not an optimal fuel for your brain. A protein bar and a cup of coffee is not the way to start your day. Make sure to eat complex carbs during the day when your body and mind are burning through fuel.

Finally, fats are more calorically dense, so they tend to make you feel heavier. Avoid fats during exercise, when you want to feel light, agile, and flexible. Additionally, fats aren't a reliably quick source of energy, so carbohydrates are a better choice during exercise. In general, eat fats in moderation to boost satiation and stave off hunger in times of lower energy expenditure, but limit them at most other times of day.

All In the Timing

That's my basic strategy for when to consume each of these macronutrients. Simple carbs during or immediately after exercise; complex carbohydrates during working hours; protein throughout the day, but not as a substitute for carbs; fats in the evening when energy expenditure lessens. Here's that info in a handy table, including a few examples:

Morning	Higher carbohydrate intake (including limited high-GL carbs) and a quickly digested protein after my morning workout to fuel the muscle-building process.	Protein shake after workout; then a bowl of oatmeal with a Tbsp of maple syrup and 1/2 cup of fried egg whites over spinach.
Afternoon	Balance of complex carbs for sustained energy, protein to meet my daily needs, and maybe a small amount of fat to help me feel full.	Grilled chicken breast over kale, and a cup of brown rice for lunch. Hard-boiled eggs, then rice cakes and peanut butter for snacks.
Evening	High in protein and low in carbohydrates. Limited fats to help me feel full.	Salmon and veggies for dinner, and then a protein shake and nuts at least an hour before bed.

TOTAL DAILY MACRONUTRIENT PERCENTAGES

The *when* of each of these macronutrients will also determine *how much* of each we need. The right macro balance will differ for each individual based on their physiology and activity levels. We all have different metabolisms, so there is no single macro split that will work for everyone all the time.

Again, do not take this to mean that you're a person who "doesn't need carbs." Most people function best when they consume a healthy variety of all three macro groups. Unless you have a medically diagnosed condition, you don't need to eliminate any one of these crucial macronutrients to achieve fat loss.

Guidelines in the United States

The Institute of Medicine indicates the following ranges as a starting point for determining a daily macronutrient balance in *Dietary Reference Intakes: The Essential Guide to Nutrient Requirements.**

---

* This information is available as part of the *Dietary Guidelines for Americans: 2015–2020*, and you can download a free copy of the report at health.gov/dietaryguidelines/2015/guidelines.

Gender, Age	Male, 19–50	Female, 19–50
Avg. calorie level assessed	2,371	1,873
Carbohydrate	45–65%	45–65%
Protein	10–35%	10–35%
Fat*	20–35%	20–35%

Total saturated fat should comprise <10% of dietary calories

These ranges are intended for "active individuals." [41] That doesn't mean *professional athletes*, it merely means that you don't spend all day on the couch. These ranges provide a starting point for calculating the percentage of each macronutrient you plan to consume each day. It's not gospel truth, but it does indicate that **the bulk of your calories should come from carbohydrates.**

My "Working" Macros

Here is my base macronutrient breakdown for days that I exercise, which includes strength training, cardio, or both:

Carbohydrates: 45%   Protein: 35%   Fat: 20%

I call those my *working macros* because I follow these numbers on days I work out. *Get it?* I prioritize carbohydrates on days I'm training because I need that energy. I work out in the morning, so I emphasize carbs at that time, and then progressively switch to favoring protein and fat as the day goes on.

My "Resting" Macros

On the days I don't exercise, I limit carbohydrates because I don't need as many of them. I never eliminate carbs entirely, but I only eat what I anticipate needing for energy during the day.

My resting day macro split looks something like this:

Carbohydrates: 20%   Protein: 50%   Fat: 30%

That's my macro split, but it might not serve you. Experiment with your macro balances to determine what works for your lifestyle and training schedule. The specific time of day isn't the important factor here. What matters is the activity you do at that time. For example, you might be someone who exercises in the evening, so you'll need carbs later in the day. If you run five miles at 9 p.m., then you will need carbohydrates at that time to fuel your activity.

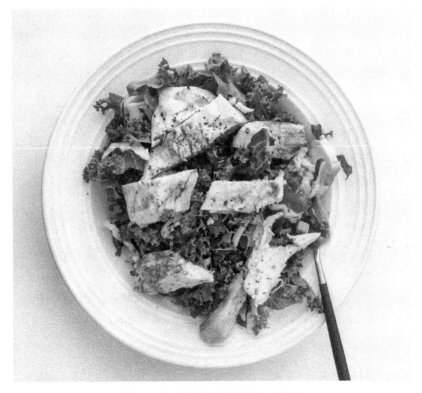

A low-carb salad with grilled chicken and kale.

HOW TO FIGURE OUT YOUR PERSONAL MACRO SPLIT

If you want a generic way to begin planning your macro split, start with your protein requirement. The United States Recommended Dietary Guidelines suggest a minimum of 5½ oz equivalent of protein per day at the 2,000 calorie/day level.[42] However, every trainer I know suggests you should consume at least 0.6 to 0.8 grams of protein per pound of body weight when trying to increase muscle mass or strength. Many bodybuilders and elite athletes argue that 1 to 1.2 grams of protein per pound is optimal for growing muscle. Many cutting programs push this number even higher (1.5 grams per pound or more) in an effort to prevent muscle loss.

I think one gram of protein per pound of body weight is a great target, especially if you are strength training. One gram per pound is also an easy number to remember because it's the same as your weight. Consider planning the amount of protein you need based on this target, and then add carbohydrates to support your activity level and energy needs throughout the day. Then add fats to balance out your total caloric needs and lifestyle.

Don't sacrifice carbohydrates and fats altogether. A high-protein, low-carb diet can indeed help you lose weight in the short term, but it's hard as hell to maintain in the long term for the following reasons:

- Protein doesn't provide the energy needed for exercise, meaning you will drag during your workouts.

- It's difficult to consume enough protein to meet your caloric needs (i.e., your BMR at a minimum).

- Protein is hard to transport because it spoils quickly.

- Some proteins make you gassy because they are harder to digest.

- Plus, protein can be *expensive*. Eating lean meats all day will break the bank. Who wants to be tired and poor?

One Size Does Not Fit All

There is no perfect, one-size-fits-all formula for how much of each macro you should eat. But guess what? That's okay because the macro split you choose is far less important than meeting your caloric deficit.

Also, it's impossible to hit your target percentages perfectly. You can use MyFitnessPal and nutrition labels to estimate the macronutrients included in the foods you consume, but you will never be 100% accurate unless you're using a spectrometer and an electron microscope or something like that. Take heart in knowing that calculating your deficit is way more crucial than perfect macro percentages. You will be successful if you stick to an appropriate deficit.

Again, when I'm trying to lose fat I vary my daily macro percentages between working (exercise) days and rest days. Maybe you were hoping that I would tell you right now exactly what you should eat each day, but that would be impossible. I don't know you. I don't know what an average workday looks like for you. I don't know how well you sleep. I don't know if you're allergic to garlic.

How could I recommend the perfect macro split without also telling you when and how much to work out each day? If I were to tell you those things, you'd most likely quit after a week or two. I'm not you. We have different needs and schedules.

Use Your Secondary Fitness Goals to Inform Your Macro Split

Assuming that your first goal is to burn fat, the macro split you choose might depend on a secondary fitness goal (e.g., muscle gain, increased energy levels, better sleep). It also depends largely on your schedule. Life is messy, so remember that this macro split business isn't an exact science.

If, for example, you know you only have time to work out three times per week, then you might only consume high-GL carbs on those days. You can eat fruit after your workout, and then avoid simple sugars on rest days, when you don't need them.

If you regularly hit the gym in the evening, you might consider limiting fats to earlier in the day to help you feel full through the afternoon, but lighter before you get to the gym. Then you might eat carbs before your workout, even though it's later. (However, I recommend limiting carbs for two hours before you go to bed.)

Here are a few suggestions for developing a macro split based on various secondary fitness goals.

GOAL: Build (or Maintain) as Much Muscle as Possible While Still Losing Fat

Building muscle while in a deficit is impossible for most people because you have less energy coming in than going out. It can happen if your deficit is small or if you are new to strength training, because your muscles experience a new stimulus and your metabolism adjusts to aid muscle growth as a consequence of that new stimulus.

If you've been training to some extent over the years, you should focus on holding on to the muscle you already have while maintaining a deficit. (Don't expect to gain muscle mass while in a deficit.) Protein intake is critical to preserve muscle when restricting calories. Consider a slightly higher protein intake, maybe even a larger percentage of protein than carbohydrates.

Check the mirror and measure your body composition in target muscle groups. Changes in size in specific areas of your body may be due to muscle loss. You don't want that, and increasing protein intake is a partial insurance policy against it.

GOAL: To Walk a 5K with Your Family

I'm a big advocate for making strength training the number one exercise component of your fat-loss strategy, but I realize that some people have other goals that might benefit from a different approach. Maybe you want to run a half-marathon to honor your mom's fight against breast cancer. Maybe you want to be able to walk around the block with your wife and kids in the evening without feeling exhausted. If your secondary fitness goal revolves around a cardiovascular form of exercise (e.g., walking, running, cycling, swimming), then consider a slightly higher carbohydrate percentage in your macro split.

You will need quick-burning, readily accessible energy to fuel cardio workouts. Don't go crazy—especially with sugar—and remember that the caloric deficit must be your priority if you want to lose fat. For instance, don't drink a Gatorade after a long run if it's going to put you outside your deficit. Again, this is why food planning is critical: if you know you've got an intense cardio workout coming up, plan your carb intake around it. Listen to your body, learn from how you feel with each workout, and adjust your macro split accordingly.

GOAL: Better Sleep, More Energy... or Something Else

Some people sleep better with a carb-heavy dinner. Others do not. No matter what anyone tells you (studied or otherwise), only you know how certain macronutrients affect your body in different scenarios. I know for myself that simple carbs on an empty stomach cause my blood sugar to spike beyond comfortable limits, ultimately throwing me into an energy spiral. So I consume high-GL carbs immediately after a fasted workout, when I know my blood sugar is low and I need a rebound.

But maybe you wake up exhausted and need a piece of fruit to get yourself to the gym. Maybe you're trying to give up caffeine and you need a quick boost. Or maybe you know that you relax and sleep better if you eat something sweet in the evening. (Still, stopping carbs two hours before bed is best.)

It wouldn't be fair for me to tell you that you're wrong… because I'm not you. All I can do is remind you to listen—*really pay attention*—to your body and adjust according to the way you feel. If a macro plan doesn't work for you, scrap it and try something else.

Try a Split Based on Your Goals and See If It Works

I've presented you with several possibilities for determining a macro plot for your lifestyle. Remember that there is no one-size-fits-all formula for determining how much of each macronutrient you should consume. *You need them all.* You also need some more than others at specific times, based on what you are doing.

Before you commit to a macro split, consider how much you're moving, when you are moving, and what your secondary fitness goals are. As long as you maintain a caloric deficit you will lose weight. Use the macro split to fine-tune your energy needs throughout the day.

Your macronutrient balance will change based on your schedule, when you work out, your ability to food prep, etc. Food planning becomes essential the more intent you are on discovering which macro split works best for you. If you plan your food ahead of time based on the kind of day you anticipate, you will minimize surprises and give yourself a better chance of learning which macro splits support your life. After a few months of committed food planning and journaling, you will have an accurate picture of how different foods affect you.

Once you've committed to a macronutrient balance or a weekly macro split, you'll be able to roll with the punches, as they say. You can approach your daily food requirements based on the *IIFYM* method.

THE IIFYM APPROACH

IIFYM is an acronym that stands for: **If It Fits Your Macros**. IIFYM means, in essence, that you can eat whatever the hell you want *if* it fits your macronutrient goals.

Once you decide on a macronutrient split that works for your goals, you should eat around that split each day. Schedule your meals to hit your target percentages, and then track those percentages throughout the day so that you know your balance of carbs, protein, and fats. Food planning around a macro split is more about planning for the percentages than it is about planning the food you'll eat. If you follow an IIFYM plan, then you can change things up on the fly—when the shit hits the fan—while staying within your macro split.

IIFYM is the secret to staying flexible while achieving your goals. You plan your meals, but then you roll with the punches when those meals are thrown out of whack, which will happen to you because it happens to everyone.

Let's walk through a scenario that happened to me last week:

Nate's Terrible, Awful, No Good (For His Diet) Day

3 a.m.

My day starts when my dog, Viola, wakes up with diarrhea. Something she ate? Who knows… but I can't get back to sleep because she is crying all night (except for when I'm standing outside with her as she's pooping). *I will be tired today*, I think, *probably moody, and it's gonna be hard to focus.*

5 a.m.

I can't stay in bed, pretending to sleep anymore. Viola is messed up, so I need to take her to the vet when they open at seven. That means I can't go to the gym this morning before work. Typically, I exercise first thing in the morning, in a fasted state. Then I drink a post-workout shake, followed by a meal with a 50-40-10 split of carbs-protein-fat an hour later. But I can't work out this morning because my dog needs me! Those carbs will be wasted (or stored) if I eat them without exercising. Instead of a carb-heavy breakfast, I adjust my morning macro split and eat something higher in protein and fat. Perhaps that's two hard-boiled eggs over kale. I limit the carbs until later when I plan to hit the gym.

12 p.m.

Viola is okay. I've been at my desk for a few hours, and it's time to squeeze in a workout on my lunch break. I know that if I eat before I lift I will feel bloated and heavy. *No, thanks!* So, I drink a branched-chain amino acid (BCAA) mix (to ensure that I have some free branched-chain aminos floating in my system to support endurance, muscle growth, and muscle recovery) and then head to the gym on an empty stomach.

1:15 p.m.

I finished my workout and I'm back at my desk. Now comes a moment I can eat lunch while I'm working. It's an excellent time for carbs because I've depleted my glycogen stores. My macros for this meal mimic my typical morning balance: 50-40-10. This might look like chicken, brown rice, spinach, and maybe half a handful of almonds.

The Rest of the Day

And now I'm back on track. I'll be at my desk until 5 p.m., then home for dinner. So, what do my macro percentages look like for the rest of the day? I'm a little off-balance, and my routine has been out of whack. However, I've been tracking my food and my macros, so I know exactly how much of each macro I need to eat in order to hit my targets at the end of the day.

This is why tracking and planning is so important… because it sets you up for success when life throws you off track. If you track your calories and plan your meals, you have a template that you can shuffle around when shit hits the fan.

Again, you don't plan your meals so you can be *perfect all the time*. You aren't tracking so that you can shame yourself when you have an impromptu slice of the birthday cake that someone brought to the office for Jessica's birthday.

You plan and track to know where you are at any given point in the day. That allows you to adjust on the fly and make good decisions based on expecting the unexpected.

If you know what you've eaten today or expect to eat later, then you can eat the unexpected thing in front of you *if it fits your macros*.

Does that slice of Jessica's birthday cake fit your macros? Then go for it.

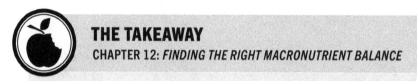

THE TAKEAWAY
CHAPTER 12: *FINDING THE RIGHT MACRONUTRIENT BALANCE*

Maintaining a caloric deficit is always more important than your macro split. *Always*.

Your body needs all three macronutrients to stay in balance. Don't follow a diet that eliminates or severely limits a macronutrient group, unless your doctor recommends it.

Timing matters:

» Favor simple carbohydrates for energy during exercise, and in your post-workout meals to provoke the insulin response.

» Favor complex carbohydrates throughout the day to sustain energy without causing radical swings in blood sugar levels.

» Favor protein at times of less energy expenditure, such as while sitting at your desk or while watching television.

» Use fats sparingly to help you feel full between meals. Consider adding healthy fats, such as a handful of nuts, as a final evening snack.

I aim for different macro percentages based on days I work (exercise) and days I rest. I explain this in greater detail in the following chapter, but here are my baseline percentages:

» **Nate's "working" macros:** 45% carbohydrate, 35% protein, 20% fat

» **Nate's "resting" macros:** 50% protein, 30% fat, 20% carbohydrate

Consider your energy requirements, how much rest you get, and your secondary goals when targeting macronutrient percentages. *There is no "one-size-fits-all" solution.*

Plan your macro split ahead of time by outlining your meals for the day (e.g., with the help of a food journal). Then, use the **IIFYM** method based on what you've eaten or planned for the future. This way, you will have flexibility in hitting your target macro split for the day, no matter what surprises throw you off.

CHAPTER 13

THE MACRO/DEFICIT SPLIT
FOR FAT LOSS

Tomorrow belongs to those who can hear it coming.

DAVID BOWIE

A WEEKLY APPROACH TO YOUR DEFICIT & MACROS

So far we've covered how your body utilizes various macronutrients and how you should emphasize them at different times based on your activities:

Carbohydrates are good for energy and for provoking the insulin response. Time them to coincide with workouts—both strength training and cardio—and at times when you need energy. (This includes office hours.)

Protein builds muscle. Consume quick-digesting proteins immediately post-workout, and spread the balance of protein throughout the day. Aim for one gram of protein per pound of body weight.

Fat is calorically dense, which means it has lots of calories. Use it sparingly to stave off hunger, and to balance your energy levels.

Knowing when to prioritize each macronutrient helps you to avoid spikes and dips in energy and mood. To lose weight, you must restrict your calories and create a caloric deficit, but that doesn't mean you need to be hungry all the time. *Far from it.*

Being hungry provokes the starvation response and will probably ruin your mood too. Being tired or grumpy makes it difficult to achieve your goals. Constant hunger will sabotage your plans, and eating at or near your BMR will probably make you hungry. Hunger may especially be problematic if you're accustomed to eating twice your daily caloric requirements.

So how do you create a significant caloric deficit without being hungry all the time? Allow me to introduce the *macro/deficit split*:

> **A macro/deficit split is the practice of varying your caloric deficit targets and your macro targets each day based on whether you exercise or rest.**

Part 1: The (Caloric) Deficit Split

As the name suggests, a caloric deficit split varies the caloric deficit you shoot for based on your activity level for the day. You set a goal deficit for the *week*, and then divide it up day-by-day depending on whether you plan to exercise or not. **Large deficits on rest days and small ones on training days.** You eat more comfortably on the days you train—when you need the energy—and restrict your calories more on the days you rest.

Large deficits are close to your BMR.

Small deficits might only be 100 or 200 calories below your TDEE.

Medium deficits fall somewhere between these two.

Let's use a 4-day training split as an example. A 4-day split is an excellent approach to weight training while burning fat. I've also indicated HIIT training on some of these days. I will explain both of these things later in the book. With a 4-day split, your week looks something like this:

Monday: Strength Training

Tuesday: Strength Training & HIIT

Wednesday: Rest

Thursday: Strength Training

Friday: Strength Training & HIIT

Saturday & Sunday: Rest *(maybe adding some long, slow cardio, like a three-mile walk to the park with your family)*

How might you approach nutrition throughout the week with a schedule like this? You know you need to favor carbohydrates on days you exercise. If you neglect carbohydrates on those days, you will be tired and you may forfeit muscle gains. You'll be hungry, and it will be even harder to do it again the next day. Therefore, *it's dangerous to attempt larger caloric deficits on training days.*

But what about rest days? Rest days—the days when you aren't strength training or doing cardio—are well suited for larger caloric deficits. Maximizing your caloric deficit on rest days benefits you in the following ways:

- You aren't exercising, so your caloric needs are lower and you're less hungry, which means you will naturally eat less.

- You've increased your deficit on days when your total energy expenditure is lower, therefore decreasing the risk of the starvation response.

- If your body does enact the starvation response on a day that your deficit is large, you can "trick" it the following day (or the day after that) by increasing your calories on a training day. This way, your body knows that there is food to be had, and your hormones, mind, and body are less likely to make you fall off the wagon.

Your body needs more calories on the days that it burns more calories. That's enough information to support increasing your caloric deficit on days you don't train. Using the 4-day training split above, and assuming a 3,500-calorie deficit for a loss of one pound of fat per week, you might cut calories with the following approach:

Monday: Strength Training — *medium deficit*

Tuesday: Strength Training & HIIT — *small deficit*

Wednesday: Rest — *large deficit*

Thursday: Strength Training — *medium deficit*

Friday: Strength Training & HIIT — *small deficit*

Saturday: Rest — *large deficit*

Sunday: Rest — *large deficit*

Determine which days you require more calories for exercise, and to what extent those days impact your overall goals. You may find you can't cut calories at all on days with cardio because you are exhausted—*and that's okay!* The most vital thing is to **target a specific total caloric deficit for the entire week, and then make daily choices to support that target.** It doesn't have to happen every day.

Don't make it harder to meet your goals by fighting for large deficits every single day of the week. *Don't be a hero.* Spread it around based on your activity levels. Create a larger deficit on days when you rest. The body responds to a caloric deficit by storing fat or limiting the metabolic process to conserve energy. As such, it makes sense that this should happen on rest days when the total stress on your system is lower.

Part 2: The Macro Split

The other part of the macro/deficit split is... *you probably guessed it...* the macro split. As presented earlier, this is a way to organize the intake of your macronutrient percentages based on the activities you do each day. It's a useful tool for strength training while trying to lose fat. Just remember that the macro part of this macro/deficit split is secondary to the caloric deficit you plan to achieve each week. Without a solid caloric deficit, you won't lose the fat.

You know the caloric values and functions of the three essential macronutrients, so it should be obvious how to favor certain macronutrients on days of exercise and cut them on days of rest. In particular, there is one macronutrient you should reserve for training days...

I'm talking about carbohydrates, the quick-energy, insulin-provoking, wonder-macro. **You should limit carbohydrates on rest days.**

Why, you ask? Carbs are the macro that is most easily stored as fat. If you consume them but don't burn them off with an activity like strength training or cardio, your body will likely save them for another day by placing them in a sack on your belly.

Carbs on rest days are especially dangerous when combined with a larger deficit because your body approaches starvation mode on those days. If your body thinks that hard times are coming because you aren't eating as much, it will store those carbs as fat to get through said troubled times. You're also likely to crave sugary foods, and God knows it's very easy to find those when you want them.

**Prioritize carbs on days when you train,
and limit them on days you don't.**

Conversely, you know that fat and protein are more filling—particularly fat. So you also know that favoring those macronutrients on high-deficit days will help you to feel fuller longer and, theoretically, convince your body that everything is copacetic. *Make sense?*

**Prioritize protein and add a little more fat on days with
larger caloric deficits. Limit fats on days you train.**

I swear to you that this kind of macro/deficit split will help you maintain a caloric deficit without being crazed by hunger. Instead of attempting a challenging deficit that becomes increasingly harder to maintain, implement larger deficits on days of rest and give your body all the nutrients it needs, when it needs them, on days you train.

If you think about it, *our bodies are built to work this way.* Use food as a tool to support the activities your body performs, and you will crush your fitness goals.

THE MACRO/DEFICIT SPLIT IN PRACTICE

Here's how the macro/deficit split might play out in the 4-day strength-training split example above. The goal in this example is still to lose one pound of fat per week. One pound of fat still equals 3,500 calories, so my total deficit for the week must be 3,500 calories.

On rest days, when energy expenditure is naturally lower, I can get close to my BMR without provoking the starvation response. My present BMR is 1,700 calories[*] and I don't ever want to eat less than that, so I'll plan to consume 1,750 calories on rest days. My rest day TDEE is 2,400 calories, so I'll use that as a starting point:

2,400 calories (TDEE) – 1,750 calories consumed (just above my BMR)
= **650-calorie deficit on rest days**

---

[*] I know I indicated a BMR of 1,648 calories earlier in the book, but I put on a bit of muscle since then!

Assuming I can maintain a 650-calorie deficit on rest days, those days contribute 1,950 calories to my total weekly deficit:

650 calories x 3 days of rest (Wed, Sat, Sun) = **1,950-calorie deficit**

That means I must trim a total of 1,550 calories on my four training days, creating training day deficits as follows:

1,550 calories / 4 (exercise days) = **387.5-calorie deficit per day**

With this approach, I'll consume approximately 164 calories more on days when I train than on days when I rest. That might not seem like a huge difference, but **it's a 25% reduction in the size of my daily caloric deficit**. Considering that if I run for 15 minutes at six miles per hour (i.e., a 10-minute mile), I burn approximately 186 calories,[43] you can see how I traded that exercise on an active day for a larger caloric deficit on a rest day. It's all about balancing calories in to calories out.

My Weekly Caloric Intake, Based on This Deficit Split

Monday: Training — 1,912 calories

Tuesday: Training + HIIT — 1,912 calories

Wednesday: Rest — 1,750 calories

Thursday: Training — 1,912 calories

Friday: Training + HIIT — 1,912 calories

Saturday: Rest — 1,750 calories

Sunday: Rest — 1,750 calories

You might decide to begin by calculating the calories you need on training days, and then divvy up the remaining weekly caloric deficit among your rest days. If your training day deficit leaves you sluggish and starved, you should *decrease* the deficit on those days and increase it further on rest days. As long as you don't eat below your BMR, you'll be fine.

All of these numbers are merely examples, and of course your plan depends on your daily TDEE. That changes based on the types of exercise you do, how often you exercise, as well as your general daily activity levels. But, with a plan such as this—creating a caloric deficit by eating less, as opposed to doing more cardio—these numbers can get you where you want to go in a safe, sustainable way.

Remember that rest days may come in many forms, and sometimes rest days are unexpected. Vacations, holidays, travel days, or even injuries often *force* you to take a rest day. The common cold might turn your regular Tuesday chest day into a rest day. I plan my deficit split based on my *anticipated* activity for each day of the week, but I adjust as things come up.

Remember: eat for the activity you are doing <u>today</u>, not merely because it's Tuesday and on Tuesdays you *eat big*.

How This Looks With Macros

Now let's add the macro details to this split (carbohydrates, protein, and fats indicated as percentages of "c/p/f" in the list below). Using the sample 4-day split week above, I favor carbohydrate intake on days when my body needs energy, and I favor protein and fat on rest days. (The following example builds on the *working* and *resting* macro splits I outlined in the previous chapter.)

Monday: Training — 1,912 calories — 45c/35p/20f

Tuesday: Training + HIIT — 1,912 calories — 50c/30p/20f

Wednesday: Rest — 1,750 calories — 20c/50p/30f

Thursday: Training — 1,912 calories — 45c/35p/20f

Friday: Training + HIIT — 1,912 calories — 50c/30p/20f

Saturday: Rest — 1,750 calories — 20c/50p/30f

Sunday: Rest — 1,750 calories — 20c/50p/30f

Notice that the carb percentages I've shown here are slightly higher on days I do HIIT (cardio), and fall somewhere around 50% of my daily macronutrient breakdown. HIIT requires quick-burning carbohydrates because glycogen stores deplete rapidly when you sprint on the treadmill, bike, etc. I need those extra carbs to replenish glycogen in my muscles. HIIT days might also be the days I choose to increase my sugar consumption to help regulate blood sugar levels. Natural sugars only, and in moderation of course. I might do this with a piece of fruit immediately following the HIIT session. (Much more info about HIIT and cardio in general in Part Four.)

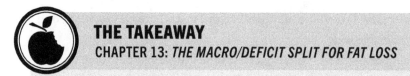

THE TAKEAWAY
CHAPTER 13: *THE MACRO/DEFICIT SPLIT FOR FAT LOSS*

The solution for optimizing calories based on activity is called a **macro/deficit split**. You alternate your caloric and macronutrient intake throughout the week based on your daily energy requirements:

» Aim for a larger caloric deficit on rest days, when activity is lower, and smaller caloric deficits on days when you train.

» Prioritize carbohydrates on training days. They will provide the energy your body needs during exercise and muscle building.

» Limit carbohydrate intake on rest days; otherwise, your body may be inclined to store those excess carbs as fat.

» Prioritize protein and fat on rest days when your body burns less energy.

» Increase fat on rest days—when your caloric deficit is greater—to feel more "full" while still limiting your calories.

How to Create a Macro/Deficit Split:

» Determine your total target caloric deficit for the entire week;

» Assume that your rest day deficit will be at or just above your BMR. Multiply your BMR by the number of rest days;

» Subtract the total caloric deficit of all rest days from your total target caloric deficit for the week;

» Divide the remaining caloric deficit between your training days. Tweak the macronutrient percentages on rest days based on how you feel while exercising.

Create your macro/deficit split based on realistic goals, including the other factors that may increase or decrease your energy expenditure, i.e., life stuff.

Don't be afraid to adjust these splits based on your progress week-over-week! Your goal is to maintain a healthy deficit over time without provoking the starvation response. Don't settle for feeling tired and hungry.

CHAPTER 14

BULKING VS. CUTTING

I didn't mean to gain weight.
It happened by <u>snaccident</u>.

UNKNOWN

"Bulking" and "cutting" are two popular terms you might hear as you spend more time among gym bros. Each strategy entails a different approach to nutrition and strength training, with *bulking* implying a weight-gaining phase and *cutting* implying a fat-loss phase. The meaning behind each word seems obvious, but the tactics people apply to achieve them are complex and varied.

So, what are the differences, and how do they fit into the strategy I propose in this book? I'm about to tell you.

BULKING

Bulking implies a training phase or program in which the goal is to gain more muscle. "Isn't that always the goal?" you may ask. *Yes and no.*

Weight training is, of course, a means to tax your muscles and thereby stimulate strength and growth. However, building muscle comes with a price for most people: *adding fat.* Why? We've established that the key to fat loss is creating a caloric deficit (i.e., burning more calories than you consume). The opposite holds for gaining muscle: your body must be in a caloric *surplus* to increase muscle mass.

You cannot gain muscle mass without more energy going toward that mass. For most people this means that you need to *eat more* to build muscle. The more muscular you are, the more metabolically tuned you already are, and the harder it becomes to gain even more muscle. You need to create a caloric surplus to gain muscle, and a caloric surplus is the *opposite* of a caloric deficit.

Hence the "bulking" phase of a training regimen, where you prioritize an increase in mass over a decrease in fat.

Bulking: a training cycle in which priority is given to muscle building, necessitating a caloric surplus without attempting fat loss.

Some people can gain muscle mass while simultaneously losing fat, but that's rare. It may happen when someone trains for the first time because their bodies learn to process calories in a new way by feeding muscles that they've previously neglected. If you experience muscle growth while also losing fat, it's the result of one or more of the following:

a. A redistribution of the way your body burns calories, most often by metabolizing calories more efficiently to build muscle while also losing fat;

b. A genetic predisposition for very efficient fat metabolism, allowing you to metabolize higher amounts of fat for energy without reducing calories; or,

c. You're confused about exactly how many calories you consume versus how many calories you burn.

However it happens, the total net caloric equation still applies: you need calories to build muscle. If you eat less, are losing fat, and are also gaining muscle mass, there is still a surplus of energy being used for muscle growth. You are either consuming that surplus, or your body is redefining the way it metabolizes the calories you eat.

How Bodybuilders Do It

Here's something you might not know: many bodybuilders, fitness models, and athletes spend a large portion of their year in a bulking cycle. And they get *fat*. The pictures you see of fitness models are not how those people look year-round, and certainly not how they look when trying to increase muscle mass.

During those bulks, they try to gain as much muscle as possible without paying so much attention to their body fat percentage. They bulk by maintaining a caloric surplus, and some of those excess calories are likely to be stored as fat.

Once they're satisfied with the increases in muscle mass, they change their approach in order to lose the extra fat they gained during the bulk. This is especially true when they have a competition or photo shoot coming up. That's when they switch to a *cutting* phase.

CUTTING

Cutting, or a "cut" phase, is a cycle that prioritizes fat loss via caloric deficit, while also trying to maintain as much muscle as possible.

Bodybuilders often start a cut a few months in advance of a competition or shoot, because they will likely lose muscle if they try to drop fat too quickly. They maintain a gentle caloric deficit while continuing to train, allowing them to lose the excess fat without sacrificing muscle. Then, after the competition or photo shoot, they switch back to a bulking cycle and attempt to gain *even more* muscle.

The cutting phase resembles everything I've mentioned thus far. It prioritizes a caloric deficit while attempting to avoid the starvation mode. There is nothing more dangerous than a hungry bodybuilder, so planning and consideration must be taken into account when they attempt a deficit. Otherwise stuff starts to break. Walls, furniture, etc.

FINDING A BALANCE

Non-professionals (like me!) can switch easily between bulking and cutting phases, too. The trick is to do so in moderation.

Even with an entirely clean diet, a caloric surplus will likely increase body fat. And the larger the surplus, the more likely that becomes. People get into trouble with bulking phases because they use the bulk as an excuse to eat whatever they want. Bulking becomes synonymous with "binging" and eating *off-plan*. That's the wrong approach.

If you're trying to bulk, you still need to follow the math. If you take a measured, mindful approach to bulking, you can limit the amount of fat you gain alongside that muscle. **You can experience muscle gains with a caloric surplus of as little as 100 or 200 calories per day.** That's a very modest surplus, and will prevent you from blowing up.

Approach a surplus the same way you approach a caloric deficit: with moderation and precision. *No, you cannot eat two pints of ice cream and an extra sirloin because you are bulking.* You can achieve size increases with a small caloric surplus. If you limit your bulk to an extra protein shake or two, the likelihood of gaining back the fat you've lost is pretty low.

Likewise, cutting is *not* an overnight starvation diet! The rule about eating above your BMR always holds, no matter your goals. Don't starve yourself after a bulking phase, or your body will catabolize muscle. The caloric deficit in a "cut" operates the same way it does during any other fat-loss endeavor: with precision and mindfulness. Either of these approaches takes time.

Each Approach Requires Some Sacrifice

If you want to gain muscle, you will probably have to gain some fat. If you want to reduce your body fat percentage, you will likely lose some muscle mass. However, if you act in moderation, you limit the chance of the unwanted consequences of either approach.

You are genetically predisposed to gain or lose fat and muscle in specific percentages based on your genes, your BMR, and the amount of training you do. Learn how your body balances energy in and out, and then set goals based on your personal experience—*not based on what anyone else is doing*.

So, What's Your Goal?

A few genetically gifted people can eat whatever they want and turn it into muscle. Unfortunately for us mortals, we must choose *one primary goal*: either to burn fat or to gain muscle. It's doubtful that both will happen simultaneously, and hoping for that miracle only leads to frustration.

Losing Fat

If you are reading this book, then I assume your primary goal is to burn excess fat. The entire concept of maintaining a caloric deficit mirrors a cutting approach. Cutting calories helps you get the lean, muscular look you want. Everything I've presented in this book so far will help you lose fat.

Most people won't gain muscle while in a caloric deficit, but a lean physique typically looks (and feels) more muscular anyway. Cutting is a fantastic approach if you want to feel good at the beach this summer—when you know you'll be taking your clothes off. Personally, I also *feel* better with a lower body fat percentage, even if I'm not carrying as much muscle mass. I like to be light and nimble in case someone is chasing me. Just kidding. *Wait—is someone chasing me?!*

Gaining Muscle

However, maybe you're happy with the way your jeans fit and you want to focus on gaining muscle now. That's great! You won't stay as lean, but you will fuel your body so that it can grow.

Create a small caloric surplus and track how your body gains muscle over several weeks and months. Start with your estimated TDEE, and add 100 to 300 calories of excess calories each day. Keep these additional calories within your target macronutrient goals. Don't limit them to protein, carbs, or fat. Beginners might hope to increase their muscle mass by approximately 0.75% of their body weight each week, while seasoned lifters might only experience increases of 0.25% or less. That's not much, so don't fool yourself into thinking you'll gain lots more muscle by overeating. Don't binge, and don't use this cycle as an excuse to eat whatever you want. If your macros shift out of balance, you are likely going to gain excess fat.

During a bulk, most professionals I've spoken to limit their maximum body fat percentage to 15%, which is a healthy percentage for most people. Once they hit 15%, they shift back toward a caloric deficit.

Don't Be Afraid to Switch It Up

The good news is that you can alternate between bulking and cutting throughout the year. That's a great way to mix up your fitness goals and to push yourself in new directions. The critical thing to remember is that you should pick one goal at any given time, either fat loss or muscle gain, and act accordingly. *Don't expect to be able to do both at the same time.*

If you know what you're reaching for, you can focus on it without being rattled by the unwanted side effects of either approach. Maintain focus on your primary goal, and remember that you can always switch gears if you need to.

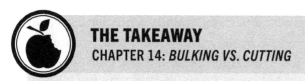

THE TAKEAWAY
CHAPTER 14: *BULKING VS. CUTTING*

Bulking is a training cycle in which you prioritize an increase in muscle mass over fat loss. Gaining muscle requires a caloric surplus for most people. A side effect of a bulking phase is an increase in body fat.

Cutting is a training cycle in which you prioritize fat loss over increases in muscle mass. Losing fat requires a caloric deficit. A side effect of a cut is a loss of some muscle mass.

Bulking is not an excuse to eat whatever you want, whenever you want. Bulking is not a synonym for "binging." You can accomplish a bulk with a small caloric surplus of as little as 100 additional calories daily. The more calories you consume as a surplus of your TDEE, the more likely you are to store those calories as fat.

Cutting is not an excuse to starve yourself. This book focuses on how to maintain a *healthy* caloric deficit, and those rules still apply when you are already somewhat lean and muscular. A cut is never an excuse to eat below your BMR. The starvation response leads to a loss of muscle mass, either via a decrease in metabolic rate, muscle catabolism (your body breaking down your muscles for energy), or because you're just too damn tired to lift. The smaller your caloric deficit, the less likely your body is to lose muscle.

If you decide to bulk, then your objective should be to increase muscle mass while minimizing fat gain. You can only hope to gain between 0.25% and 0.75% of your body weight in muscle mass per week, so anticipate that slow growth. Many professionals tend to limit their maximum body fat percentage to 15% while bulking.

If you decide to cut, then your objective should be to lose body fat while maintaining as much muscle mass as possible. Calculate a safe deficit based on precisely how much fat you'd like to lose in a reasonable amount of time.

Switch between bulking and cutting throughout the year in order to pursue different goals. But **pick one approach at a time**: either train to lose fat or train to build muscle. Don't expect to achieve both simultaneously, because that's impossible for most people. You'll only get frustrated... and frustration often results in abandoning your goals.

CHAPTER 15

EATING CLEAN

Where then do I look for good and evil? Not to uncontrollable externals, but within myself to the choices that are my own…

EPICTETUS

"CLEAN IT UP, BRO"

You've undoubtedly heard people talk about *eating clean*. You're probably wondering how eating clean compares to the IIFYM approach or if they are compatible approaches.

Time for a quick quiz: What does "eating clean" entail?

a. Eating a "fat-free" diet
b. Skipping desserts and sweets
c. Eating flavorless foods (bland, no spices)
d. Limiting foods that are processed or complicated by lots of ingredients so that you *know* what you're eating
e. Eating a vegetarian or vegan diet
f. Eating a Paleo diet

[Cue the *Jeopardy* music…]

This is a trick question. The correct answer is *d*. Many people who eat clean do so as part of a broader diet, but **those dietary restrictions are not mandatory** for clean eating. Some clean-eaters follow the other diets listed above while *also* eating clean. You can be vegetarian *or* Paleo and still eat clean. That's why it's confusing! Here's how I define eating clean:

Eating clean means being aware of what's in the food you eat, and attempting to eat foods that are as close to the three "pure" macronutrients (protein, carbohydrates, and fats) as possible.

Eating clean means that you strive to consume your macronutrients in their purest forms so that you know their caloric density and macronutrient composition to the best of your ability. That allows you to calculate your calories with as much accuracy as possible.

Eating clean is not a diet; it's a philosophy that works hand in hand with maintaining a caloric deficit and attempting any macro split. If you count calories to maintain a deficit and track your macros to maintain a specific macro split, then you must know where your calories are coming from and how much of each macronutrient is in everything you eat. How can you know the calories and macronutrients in the thing you are eating if you don't know where it came from or what's in it?

To me, eating clean means consuming food in its purest form possible. You already know that maintaining a caloric deficit is the only way to lose fat, and you also know that it's essential to count your calories so that you can calculate that deficit. Now you know that you must prioritize "eating clean" in order to have the best possible guess at exactly how many calories you consume each time you open your mouth.

Quiz #2: Which of each of the following meals is "clean"?

Pick one from each pair. The answers are at the bottom of the next page.

- a. Grilled chicken with 1 Tbsp marinara sauce and 1 Tbsp breadcrumbs
- b. Chicken parm you ordered at your favorite Italian restaurant

- a. Broccoli you sautéed in olive oil yourself
- b. A spinach salad with balsamic vinaigrette your sister made

- a. A freshly baked doughnut from the grocery store bakery
- b. A slice (serving) of a Duncan Hines cake you make from the box

That last pair is tricky. My friend Jessica just told me she considers both options to be "nutritionally awful." Be that as it may, only one of these options tells you precisely *what* you're eating. Hint: knowing is still half the battle.

Eating clean means knowing what you eat, with as much accuracy as possible, even when what you eat is—*ahem*—less than nutritionally optimal. Simple foods are easier to be certain of, but simple foods aren't always available in modern life.

Eating clean is all about knowing where your calories originate so that you can track them efficiently. By eating clean—simply, with as much specific information as possible about the macronutrient breakdown and quality of your food—you increase the accuracy of your data. By making the cleanest food choices possible, you lower the margin of error in your deficit calculations.

IT'S NOT EASY BEING CLEAN

If you're reading this book on your iPad or Kindle, then odds are you live in an industrialized nation. This means there's a significant chance that you don't farm your own food. You buy food from grocery stores, restaurants, food trucks, and the occasional vending machine.

Most of the food that's readily available to us is heavily processed. It often includes all kinds of filler ingredients, like chemical preservatives, synthetic fats, and added sugars. Even when there is a label on an item, it's tough to know the *exact* percentages of each ingredient. It's even harder to know which macronutrients have been obfuscated or, worse, made dangerous by chemical preservatives, solvents, or unnatural molecular synthesis. (I call calories made in a lab "chemicalories." *Chemical*-calories…get it?)

Part of eating clean is trying to limit superfluous ingredients from your diet, because you can't be certain of their impact on your metabolism. But that's not always possible in today's world. *You will, most likely, eat junk food on occasion.* It's tough to eat clean 100% of the time. I'd argue that it's impossible unless you are the person growing, harvesting, slaughtering, and preparing 100% of your food.

Who has time for that? *Nobody.*

---

* Answers: a, a, b

Even if you happen to be one of those 25-year-old CrossFit bros with nothing else to do besides hit the gym and then troll the farmers market for all of your vegetables, eventually you will have a job and a family and you won't have time for that shit.

Maybe you have kids, and kids like to go to Chuck E. Cheese once in a while.

Q: How do you eat clean at a Chuck E. Cheese?

A: You don't.

Maybe you typically brown-bag your lunch, but today you were running late…which means you eat lunch from the company vending machine. There's definitely nothing 100% clean in there, but you need to eat *something*.

Maybe your spouse is a terrible cook, or they just love Thai food, so you opt for takeout once in a while. *I hear that!* It happens. We try our best to eat clean, but sometimes we need to choose convenience first. When your fat-loss strategy depends on eating perfectly cleanly all the time, you set yourself up to fail. Circumstances change regularly, and we can't expect to eat whole, organic, unprocessed foods that we've weighed with meticulous precision *all the time*. Here is my philosophy:

> **Make the cleanest possible choices you can, as often as you can, and adjust your calories on days when clean eating is impossible.**

Life is too messy to expect perfection because life is not a perfectly curated salad next to a piece of trout you caught with your bare hands. So how do we cope with life's uncleanliness?

A SUSTAINABLE APPROACH TO EATING CLEAN

These are the strategies I use to stay on track, even when staying on track seems unlikely.

I Choose "Clean" Foods Whenever Possible

I pick foods in their purest form; I opt for single, unprocessed ingredients in the recipes I cook; and I prepare about 70% of the food I eat. I grill chicken in bulk, I bake salmon fillets for dinner, and I eat vegetables raw or steamed most of the time.

If I cook the chicken breast, I know I didn't put butter on it. (Unless I did, in which case I know exactly how much butter I used. *#butterybutterychicken*)

I also weigh my food on a kitchen scale as often as I can, so I know how much chicken I am consuming. I don't guess. I aim for accuracy.

That's how I know I eat clean approximately 70% of the time.

I Get Help From a Database

We've talked about the importance of tracking food so that you can calculate your deficit. Tracking in a diet app also helps you to monitor the cleanliness of your meals. Programs like MyFitnessPal include a database of food information that will calculate calories, macros, and ingredients of the foods you eat. It also helps with packaged foods because it includes a bar code scanner to read the SKUs on wrappers! You can scan the packaging and track the food's info immediately.

You can add custom recipes and divvy up servings to calculate the nutritional info in foods that you and others prepare. Let's say your mom made a pie. Ask her for the recipe, then enter the ingredients and MyFitnessPal will automatically calculate the carb, protein, and fat values. Even if the pie isn't "clean"—let's say it's got a ton of butter in it and you didn't measure the butter yourself—you can still *estimate* how much butter there is in each slice of pie.

Is MyFitnessPal a perfect system? Not by a long shot. Especially with all the dodo birds out there who insist on "correcting" recipes and uploading their own ideas of what pizza is made of.

Even though it's not perfect, *it's close enough to calculate your deficit.* If you track with a database, you'll have a relative picture of how cleanly you're eating, and you'll get the macronutrient information you need. Just remember, it only works if you use it. Aim for simple, clean foods at least 70% of the time.

But what about eating out? What do I do when I'm at a restaurant and I don't have any information about what I'm eating?

I Make an Educated Guess

If I don't have the info and the meal doesn't show up in the database, I do my best to guess while also trying to make healthy choices. I use MyFitnessPal to guess the caloric content based on similar items. Lots of restaurants print the caloric content of their meals on the menu now, so I check that first. Maybe the Marie Callender's Cobb Salad isn't in the app, but I guarantee there is one from another chain restaurant that looks similar. I'll find an item with a similar caloric value—or adjust the portion size until the calories match the calories on the menu—and presto! I have an *estimate* of the macro content for each item. It's not 100% accurate, but some info is always better than none.

There are times I'm flying in the dark. There will be snacks. There will be doughnuts at an AA meeting that don't have a nutrition label on the bright pink box. I do the best I can to guess the nutritional value of those items based on similar items, and I track my guesses. I don't pretend I didn't eat something just because I don't have the complete picture. A bad guess about the caloric content of something I just ate is always better than pretending I didn't eat it.

When I Eat Foods That Are "Unclean," I Do It With Purpose and Determination!

I own my choices, and so should you. Commit to your decisions. Don't hide from your food. Don't pretend you didn't eat something because you feel guilty about eating it.

If you want a piece of pizza, you should eat it. Live your life.

But track all of your calories, even when you go off the rails. Then course-correct with healthier choices for the rest of the day. No matter what you eat, you can always get back on track. Your next chance to make a healthy decision is coming right up. You have another opportunity to achieve your small goals each time you eat something.

If you need to splurge, then *plan* for those splurges. (More on "cheating" later in the book.) Don't give up on your goals when you make a choice you regret. *Right now* is another moment in which you have a choice about what to eat. Take the shame out of this game, and remember that it's science. Each decision is a link in the chain, and a series of good decisions will get you the results you want.

Track all the foods you eat, every day, even the meals that aren't clean. Then leverage that data. Eat as clean as possible, but remember that you are human. You exist in a world with other humans, and we all make bad decisions on the regular.

Remember that there are corporations out there fighting to profit off of your poor food choices. (Including diet peddlers!) It's challenging to say "no" when a tempting option is the only option in front of you. You're not alone in this struggle, I promise.

Do your best to eat clean, and own your decisions, even if you make a choice you'll regret later. Staying mindful about the food you choose is just as important as what you actually eat.

You control your choices, even when you don't.

FINAL THOUGHT

You'll hear lots of folks talking about eating clean, and many people have different opinions about what that means. For some, it means eating foods that are organic, free from preservatives, and locally sourced. For other people, it means eating foods that are free from added fats or added sugars. And still for others, eating clean might align with a specific diet, like avoiding grains.

Eating clean can mean all or none of these things to you. The one common thing all of these definitions share is this:

**Eating clean means knowing the
ingredients of the food you eat.**

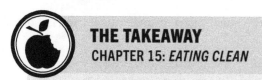

THE TAKEAWAY
CHAPTER 15: *EATING CLEAN*

I define "eating clean" as knowing the ingredients of the food you eat. Knowing what your food is made of means knowing its caloric content and macronutrient breakdown. You need to know these things in order to calculate your caloric deficit.

» Ambiguity is dirty; knowledge is power.

The simpler your foods are, the cleaner they are. Fewer ingredients mean more accuracy in knowing what your food is made of. Keep it simple by:

» Preparing your own food as often as possible;

» Striving to limit unnecessary ingredients, like added fats and sugars, chemical preservatives, or any other *chemicalories*.

Aim to eat clean at least 70% of the time.

» Track everything you eat to the best of your ability, even when you're not 100% certain of the ingredients or macros.

» If you eat something *unclean,* do it with purpose, not shame.

CHAPTER 16

FOODS I AVOID

*If trouble comes when you least expect it then maybe
the thing to do is to always expect it.*

CORMAC MCCARTHY, *The Road*

One more time for the cheap seats: the only thing you must do to lose fat is to maintain a caloric deficit. In theory, you can eat whatever you want and still lose weight. However, some foods make it *harder* for you to maintain that deficit. *Sorry!* The quality of the food you consume does impact how efficiently your body works.

Think about it like this: there are calories (energy) in dirt, but you don't eat dirt. You can see how eating dirt would cause problems in your body. It would stop you up, and it might be poisonous, etc. That's why we don't eat dirt.

Unfortunately, many of the foods we consume are as bad as dirt. It's just that we don't pay attention to how they affect us. If you eat food that disrupts the natural balance of your body, you run a higher risk of heart disease, cancer, dementia, and so on.

If you eat crappy foods, you will feel like crap. If you feel like crap, you will crave foods that make you "feel" good, like sugar, fat, and alcohol. Cravings make it harder for you to maintain your deficit. Plus, many of these foods disrupt your natural metabolic process. Metabolic dysfunction also makes it harder to maintain a deficit because you may not be burning as many calories as you might otherwise.

I already mentioned the example of the school teacher who proved that you can lose weight while eating exclusively at McDonald's. But here's what else happens when you eat a fast-food diet:

- Excess saturated fat will likely lead to an accumulation of visceral fat, even if your total body fat decreases. Scientists link this kind of fat to many other health problems, including heart disease, diabetes, and cancer.

- Excess sodium causes dehydration, which you may confuse for hunger. The salt in fast food leaves you feeling hungry so that you will crave more... and then buy more. *That's how they get ya!*

- High-fructose corn syrup—pumped into everything from buns to salad dressings—creates a spike in blood sugar. Once the spike wears off, and your blood sugar drops below average, you start to feel hungry again. This perpetuates the cycle of craving and eating. It's hard to maintain a deficit if you are always hungry.

Overall caloric intake determines weight gain or weight loss, but the quality of those calories determines how well you will be able to burn future calories. Certain foods put an unnecessary strain on my system, so I try to avoid those foods as much as possible.

With that in mind, the following is a list of the foods that I avoid:

- Added (refined) sugars
- Refined grains
- Alcohol
- Dairy products
- "Fake foods" (i.e., fake sugars and added *chemicalories*)

I know from experience that eating these foods sabotages my fitness goals. They throw me out of my caloric deficit *without* satisfying my hunger. If you cut even one of these items from your diet, you'll find it easier to maintain a deficit. Try to live without some of these foods for a few weeks and you will feel better. You'll be more in tune with your body's response to these foods, and you'll notice how these foods affect you the next time you eat them.

Nobody is perfect, but if you want to create some discipline in your diet, avoiding these foods will jump-start your goals.

ADDED SUGARS

Sugar is everywhere. No joke, I bought a can of green beans at the super-market recently, and it listed sugar as an ingredient. Who needs sugar in their green beans?

Sugar creeps into our food in myriad ways, and it takes many forms. Corn syrup, cane sugar, added fructose, glucose, sucrose… it's everywhere. I'm not going to dive deep into the political, economic, and industrial reasons that food manufacturers add unnecessary sugar to almost everything we eat, but please be vigilant and read the labels!

The Effects of Added Sugar

Added sugars wreak havoc on your body by causing unnecessary blood sugar spikes. These spikes falsify your awareness of energy expenditure, making it harder to discern actual hunger. First, you feel a rush of energy. Then, as your blood sugar dips back to lower levels, you feel tired, which makes you feel hungry again. This fluctuation in blood sugar levels is addictive, and the unnecessary insulin spikes tax your endocrine system.

Added sugars also sneak unnecessary calories into your diet. For example, a teaspoon of high-fructose corn syrup added to a cup of green beans increases the total caloric content from 44 calories to 63. *That's a 44% increase in calories.* It adds up quickly.

Manufacturers routinely add sugar to items like ketchup, yogurt, gra-nola, BBQ sauce, salad dressing, dried fruits and berries, juices, etc. The US Department of Agriculture estimates that the average American eats between 150 and 170 pounds of refined sugar each year.[44] Read the labels wrapped around the foods you buy to ensure you aren't eating more sugar than you planned for.

Synonyms for "Sugar"

Manufacturers hide added sugar under many different names. Below is a partial list of some common sugars I've seen added to food products. These sugars are "natural," but they must be harvested and refined before being added to foods that didn't initially contain them. Even though they're named differently, they are all synonyms for sugar. Check your labels, kids!

Sneaky Added Sugars:

- Beet sugar
- Brown rice syrup
- Brown sugar
- Cane sugar
- Caramel
- Confectioner's sugar
- Date sugar
- Evaporated cane juice
- Evaporated fruit juice
- Fructose
- Golden sugar
- Grape sugar
- Honey
- Lactose
- Maple syrup
- Molasses
- Muscovado sugar
- Raw sugar

Sugar for Sugar's Sake

I have a rule: if I want sugar, I eat a dessert. If I crave sugar, I'll eat candy or chocolate (in moderation, of course). Canned green beans don't need sugar! My salad doesn't need sugar added to it in the form of half a cup of sweetened cranberries. If I decide to have a Pumpkin Spice Latte, I think of that as a dessert, an occasional treat, not as something that I drink every morning before work.

When you consume refined sugar, your body triggers a specific reaction. You must understand the consequences to anticipate them. When I eat refined sugar, in any form, I feel a spike in my blood sugar level. What goes up must come down, so I "crash" when my blood sugar level swings in the opposite direction. I feel like crap when that happens.

I time sugar consumption strategically to complement my energy expenditure, e.g., I eat it right after a workout. That's the perfect time to eat natural sugars, like a piece of fruit or berries with your oatmeal. Exercise depletes glycogen reserves, so my blood sugar is already low at that point. Eating an apple after a workout brings me back to neutral. (In fact, I even add a simple carbohydrate supplement to my post-workout protein shake. *It's not an "added sugar" if I add it myself!* More on that in a later chapter.)

Many of us are addicted to sugar, and if you avoid it, you will feel better. The easiest way to avoid sugar is to make sure it's not sneaking into your foods. If you're serious about your goals, avoid foods with added sugar, and opt for naturally occurring sugars when the timing is right.

REFINED GRAINS

Foods with refined grains include bread, crackers, cakes, and the breading on the outside of a fried chicken leg. Refined grains are milled or ground up to turn them into a powder. Any grain that's been pulverized to make flour is considered a refined grain.

Refining grains makes them easier to process during industrial food preparation, and it also increases their shelf life. But when grains are refined, many valuable nutrients disappear during the process, including fiber and vitamins.

Frequently, manufacturers bleach grains during the refining process for purely aesthetic reasons. Milled grains often lighten naturally after several weeks, due to oxidation. In previous centuries oxidation happened spontaneously during storage, and it also indicated a more exceptional level of milling. Contemporary manufacturers fake this process by using chemical solvents to lighten the color. Thus, freshly milled grains have the appearance of flour that has aged naturally. *It's a scam!* **There is no nutritional or taste benefit to bleaching a grain.** On the contrary, the process further strips the product of fundamental nutrients.

I hate the idea of milling grains and then using chemicals to bleach the flour to make it white. This process turns the grain into a pure starch, which has a higher glycemic index than natural sugar. I know people who've developed type 2 diabetes late in life, despite eating what they believed to be a healthy diet. The culprit? *Bread.*

Refined grains—in the form of breads, pitas, tortillas, crackers, baked goods, etc.—impact your body the same way as sugar. Bread causes an insulin spike because there is no longer natural fiber to balance the digestive process. All that sugar goes into your system almost instantly. **There is nothing healthy about a piece of white bread.** You should think of bread as cake, even when it's savory.

> **SIDE NOTE:** When I took a weightlifting class in college, the coach explained to me how a doughnut represents the worst of the food manufacturing process. What he said really stuck with me. "They take flour, bleach it, suck out all the nutrients; they mix it with lard and sugar; then they deep fry it in more lard and coat it in more sugar," he said. Yikes.

Whole Grains Beat Refined Grains

I've previously tried to remove all grains from my diet, but it never worked for me. I did the Whole30 program,[45] and I've attempted Paleo, both of which severely limit the grains you can eat. The benefit to diets like these is that they limit your consumption of hidden sugars and chemicalories. That's a good thing. But I've also realized that my body runs better when I consume certain whole grains in moderation. These grains include rice, quinoa, and whole corn (which isn't considered a "grain" until it's dried, but might as well be).

NO BREAD, PLEASE!

In my experience, wheat is the worst possible refined grain. I avoid traditional wheat-based bread as much as possible, in all forms.

Bread consumption is associated with many other health risks in addition to diabetes. Are you familiar with the phrase *bread head*? Multiple studies have connected a high-glycemic (i.e., carbohydrate dominant) diet to Alzheimer's disease.[46] One study indicates that people with type 2 diabetes are nearly twice as likely to develop Alzheimer's.[47] As I understand it, glycemic spikes caused by ill-timed consumption of carbohydrates can weaken the body's natural ability to sweep amyloid plaque from the brain. This plaque may be a cause of Alzheimer's disease. *Does that doughnut still sound good to you?*

SIDE NOTE: The *New York Times* recently published a report chronicling the study of a woman with a rare genetic mutation that has protected her from dementia despite her having developed the major neurological features of Alzheimer's disease.[48] While this is exciting news and may open the door to therapies, it does not refute the research correlating high-glycemic diets to dementia. This particular study investigated a single person whose family has a known genetic predisposition to the disease. That example doesn't account for the 5.8 million Americans who have Alzheimer's disease. The specific causes of dementia may still be up for debate. Regardless, diets high in simple carbohydrates, like refined grains, have been linked to Alzheimer's disease.

But What If I Want a Cupcake?

If I crave cake, pie, or something else sweet, I opt for baked goods made with nut flours. These treats are more calorically dense due to the high fat content in nuts, but they don't trigger blood sugar blues the way traditional, wheat-based baked goods do. Even when a paleo cake has a lot of natural sugar in it—like coconut sugar, maple syrup, or agave—I don't experience the same spike in blood sugar as I do when I eat refined wheat. That's because bread has a higher glycemic index than table sugar.

A Kaiser roll (30g) has a glycemic index of 73 and a glycemic load of 12, while a Snickers bar (60g) has a glycemic index of 51 and a glycemic load of 15.[49] *Think about that.* Given the variation in size of store-bought Kaiser rolls along with its 41% higher GI, eating one could make your blood sugar spike higher/faster than eating a dang Snickers bar! That doesn't even account for the other food you put *inside* the roll.

I'm not advocating that you eat candy bars. But eating bread is basically the same thing. If you eat bread at every meal (e.g., rolls, buns, slices, etc.), it's akin to eating a Snickers bar with every meal. *Don't do it.* Regular bread should not be a part of your plan.

Limit Refined Grains

I eat corn off the cob, but I don't eat corn chips. I eat potato chips on occasion, but I do not eat Sun Chips.

I avoid bread. Even when it's called "whole-grain," it's actually not. If anyone tells you that a slice of whole-grain bread is healthy because of the fiber content, tell them they are wrong and remind them that you get enough fiber from fruits and vegetables.

If you want to enjoy sugar, then have sugar in its natural form. You don't need to turn wheat into sugar. If you're serious about losing fat and feeling better, skip refined grains as often as possible.

ALCOHOL

I gave up alcohol because that was a necessary, personal choice for me. I spent much of my 20s drunk to some degree, but I found help and haven't looked back.

I stopped drinking to support my mental health. My life is better now. I'm nicer, I'm less depressed or manic, and I've found that exercise is a better way to regulate my mood than alcohol ever was. I don't self-medicate, and I don't need a drink to talk to people in a crowded room. It took me many years to learn that lesson.

Later, I discovered the physiological health benefits of skipping the booze. In particular, I noticed a sharp reduction in the number of calories I consumed. Alcohol is packed with calories, and it's easy to overeat with alcohol in the following ways:

- Alcohol is liquid. Liquid calories are easier and faster to ingest without feeling "full." Those calories add up quickly.

- Alcoholic drinks are often mixed with sugary syrups and fruit juices that increase the number of calories you consume.

- Alcohol increases hunger by stimulating neurons that produce agouti-related peptide (AGrP). The brain creates this peptide during starvation mode as a way to increase appetite.

- Alcohol impairs your capacity for self-restraint; that is, it loosens inhibitions and makes it easier to cheat on your diet, among other things.

Alcohol in Moderation

I'm not trying to police all your fun! Enjoying alcohol in moderation might work for you. You might be able to consume alcohol without the adverse emotional side effects, and only you can balance the quality of calories in alcohol against your fitness goals.

If you decide you can't live without it, *seek professional help.*

If you decide you'd *rather not* live without it, consider limiting your consumption. Opt for spirits with fewer calories, and alternate alcoholic drinks with glasses of water.

Remember, those calories from alcohol count against your deficit too. A margarita is a poor choice, not only because it's high in sugar, but because the caloric content will vary wildly depending on the bartender who makes it. Gin and soda would be a safer choice because you can estimate the caloric content easily.

Regardless, if you decide to drink, track those calories in your food journal with as much accuracy as possible.

DAIRY

I love cheese. But dairy makes me gassy and bloated, so I avoid it.

Lactose is the primary sugar found in milk. Lactase is the enzyme that breaks this sugar down. In most mammals, lactase production wanes after infancy, when the offspring weans off its mother's milk and begins to eat a regular diet. Lactase most likely is only produced in adult humans as an evolutionary response to early man's discovery of dairy as a nutritional supplement. Most human adults are lactose intolerant, meaning they cannot digest it.[50] The rare ability to produce lactase as an adult is the result of a genetic mutation in response to the amount of dairy your cultural ancestors ate.[51] Europeans, for example, may have a genetic predisposition to creating lactase as adults because their cultures have been eating cheese for centuries.

In other words, your ability to digest milk depends on your cultural heritage, both racial and ethnic. It's not biologically "natural" for any of us to drink milk as adults.

The more lactose you ingest, the more likely you are to experience bloating, diarrhea, and cramping when your body can't process it. When I ate dairy, I'd often notice major differences in how different processing methods would make me feel. Certain cheeses were fine, while others made me think I was about to crap my pants. Combine that gastric stress with refined wheat (think: pizza), and I was asking my body to work with materials it isn't prepared to process. For these reasons, I avoid dairy. Mistakes happen, but I'm dairy-free for the most part.

TIP: When you eat out, ask the kitchen to cook your food with oil instead of butter. In my experience, most restaurants are willing to do this; it's often easier for a kitchen to cook with oil anyway.

"Fitness Dairy"

What about whey and casein protein powders? Aren't they milk products?

Yes, they are. Despite years of being dairy-free, I've recently been experimenting with whey and casein again.

I use whey protein in the morning after workouts because it is quick to digest, and I usually opt for whey isolate that's explicitly advertised as "lactose-free."

I also use casein protein at night before bed because it's a protein that digests slowly overnight. Our bodies build muscle during sleep, and some studies show that slow-digesting protein can help facilitate that process. Most casein products are naturally lactose-free, especially if the label says "carb-free." If there is any residual lactose in the casein products I use, it's so little that I haven't noticed any issues.

FAKE FOODS

Fake foods are foods with weird chemical ingredients that I can't pronounce. These include artificial sweeteners, bulkers, emulsifiers, and chemical preservatives... basically anything in the ingredient list with more than four syllables.

That's a broad category. As I've mentioned, I try to eat clean in the sense that I want to know the composition of the food I eat—simple foods with few ingredients.

If I can't pronounce it, I probably don't know what it's doing to my body.

With fewer fake foods in my diet, I've become more aware of how these chemicalories affect me when I do consume them. *They make me feel awful!* Symptoms range from headaches and gassiness to depression and anxiety. I had no idea these purportedly safe substitutes were wreaking havoc on my body until I eliminated them.

Fake Sugars Are Probably the Worst

There's plenty of research showing the harmful effects of artificial sugars on the body's insulin-response mechanism.[52] Fake sugar is associated with accelerated blood insulin and glucose response.[53] In other words, fake sugars destroy your ability to detect, process, and sort natural sugar as an energy source.[54] In fact, there's evidence that diet soda is worse for weight loss than regular soda.[55] At the time of this writing, the FDA has approved eight artificial and non-nutritive sweeteners for public consumption: saccharin, acesulfame-K, aspartame, neotame, sucralose, stevia, monk fruit extract, and advantame. (Please note that stevia and monk fruit extract are considered natural, but they are non-nutritive and often mixed with other sources of non-nutritive sugar.) In my opinion, the benefit of these chemicalories is overshadowed by the ways they screw with my body's natural ability to process actual sugar. I avoid them as much as possible.

As I've mentioned, if I want something sweet, I eat sugar as it was intended to be eaten: naturally occurring and in moderation. I'll have a piece of pie (made with paleo crust) that uses natural coconut sugar, maple syrup, or agave as a sweetener. I eat natural sugars, not chemical substitutes.

Even better, I'll have a piece of fruit. Most fruits have a relatively low glycemic load, because naturally occurring fructose is technically low-GI and many fruits are fibrous. (This does not apply to chemically compounded high-fructose additives.) Fructose is still a simple sugar and it will have some impact on your blood sugar level, as will *any* carbohydrate. In fact, I've also noticed that avoiding hyper-sweet fake sugars has heightened my response to fructose. An apple tastes like candy to me now. *Really!* (You probably think I'm an asshole for suggesting that an apple is the same as candy, but I'm not exaggerating.) Anyway, if you crave something sweet, always choose the fruit first.

Protein Bars Are Fake Food

I was a lacto-ovo-pescatarian for almost 13 years. (I ate fish, dairy, and eggs, but no beef, chicken, pork... you get it.) I did this primarily for health reasons. But even so, I foolishly believed that protein bars were a safe way to supplement my protein needs.

For years I would routinely eat two or more protein bars a day. Most of them were made to mimic candy bars or desserts. Even after I started to eat meat again, I continued to eat a protein bar (or four) almost every day. I had no idea those bars were tanking my fitness goals by messing with my endocrine system and forcing my body to process unnatural chemicalories.

Last year I completely cut them out. Within weeks of eliminating them from my diet, I began losing fat like never before. I'm not kidding—it was like a miracle. Even with the same caloric deficit, **something in those bars was hindering my fat-loss efforts.**

So I don't eat them. The risks outweigh the rewards. If I need protein, I eat meat, fish, poultry, and the occasional whey or casein supplement (with as few added chemicalories as possible). *I avoid protein bars.*

FINAL THOUGHT

I'm sorry if the preceding list of foods I avoid confused you or made you feel guilty about your food choices to date. That wasn't my intention. These are guidelines to consider. You do not have to survive on rabbit food to lose that fat.

Limiting these items makes a huge difference for me, and I know that it will make a difference for you, too. I don't eat perfectly all the time, and my diet is not 100% clean. I eat in restaurants. I eat packaged foods on the go. Occasionally I even eat some of the stuff on this list. Sometimes that happens by accident, and sometimes it happens because, *fuck it*, I decided to eat it! But when I do, I accept the consequences and I remain aware of how they make me feel.

**I eat with intention. I take responsibility for the
choices I make, and I don't make excuses.**

Only you can decide how far you're willing to go to meet your goals. Remember that your body is engineered to run on certain fuels: carbohydrates, proteins, and fats. You want to eat these macronutrients in their purest forms at the right times, and avoid foods that may screw up how your body processes those macros.

As you begin to lose fat and work harder to fight the starvation response, choosing foods that help your body run efficiently becomes essential for continued weight loss and maintenance. Overloading your system with crappy foods will stall your metabolism, tire you out, and make you grumpy. All of those things make it harder for you to reach your ultimate fitness goals.

You don't have to skip these foods to lose weight, but I guarantee that if you avoid the stuff on this list, you will feel better, stronger, and, overall, more aware of how your body works.

- You'll have a better perception of your insulin response and how certain foods impact your blood sugar level.
- You will feel less bloated and more regular.
- You'll be better at realizing when you are truly hungry versus thirsty or just crashing.
- And I expect that most people will notice meaningful increases in energy like I did.

All of those things happened to me when I stopped eating the foods on this list. Give it a try for a few weeks and see how you feel.

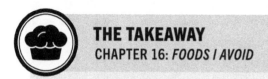

THE TAKEAWAY
CHAPTER 16: *FOODS I AVOID*

Here's a list of foods I avoid (as much as possible):

Added sugars. These sugars are added to the foods you eat, i.e., they aren't found naturally in those foods. Added sugar comes in many different forms. Check the ingredient list for hidden cane sugar, maple syrup, rice syrup, etc. Remember that this stuff shows up in the strangest places, like ketchup and canned vegetables.

Refined grains. These include any grain that's been ground up, bleached, and combined with other ingredients. Refined grains include bread, crackers, and baked goods. Stick to whole grains that are minimally processed, like rice, oats, barley, and quinoa.

Alcohol. If you want to enjoy a little booze, keep it simple: avoid fruity drinks with added sugars and syrups, and limit high-calorie beverages like beer. If you have a drink, make sure to record those calories against your deficit. Liquid calories still count, and they add up fast.

Dairy products. I avoid dairy because it makes me feel bloated and gross. As much as I like cheese, its high caloric density can tank my deficit fast. If you have regular digestive trouble, or if you struggle to maintain energy throughout the day, try giving up dairy for a few weeks and see how you feel.

Fake foods. I avoid fake sugars and chemicalories that I can't pronounce. The stranger the ingredients, the more likely that something in there will screw with my body. I watch out for high-fructose corn syrup, which is especially pervasive. If I want something sweet, I eat real, naturally occurring sugar, not chemicalories. Engineered foods are designed to be profitable for the companies that make them. They are not engineered to be nutritious or good for your body.

CHAPTER 17

TO CHEAT OR NOT TO CHEAT...

Eating crappy food isn't a reward—it's a punishment.

DREW CAREY

It doesn't matter... this is my cheat day!

How many times have you heard someone say that as they *inhaled* a pizza? Ugh. It's even worse, in my opinion, when they are in great shape. I hate watching someone with shredded abs scarf down an entire pizza. It throws me into a jealous rage.

Some people cheat as a reward for working hard. Other people believe that "cheating" makes it easier to stick to their plan later, by indulging cravings in a controlled manner. Regular cheat meals are ubiquitous among many of my friends. They eat clean all week long, then on Saturday they cut loose and mindlessly eat whatever the hell they want. Many folks who count calories during the week avoid tracking on weekends. It's as if the calories in that cheeseburger, fries, and milkshake don't count because it's Saturday night. They might even drink a few (read: many) beers and "forget" those calories too. Then they wonder why they aren't reaching their goals, even though they ignore the data right in front of them.

Guess what? **Calories always count, even on Saturdays.**

Let's start with a definition. Merriam-Webster defines the verb "cheat" as such:

> *To act dishonestly or unfairly in order to gain an advantage, especially in a game or examination; to defraud; swindle; to deceive; influence by fraud.*

How does using the word "cheat" make you feel in other contexts? In a relationship? On your taxes? It's not so cute to say, *I'm cheating!* when you think about what that actually means. I feel dishonest when I cheat, as if I'm getting something I don't deserve; like I'm unfairly gaming the system.

This book is about the simple science you need to apply to reach your goals. There are no cute shortcuts. You can't cheat physics. Energy in must be less than energy out. You cannot pretend that something you ate doesn't count toward your goals just because it's a special day, or you need to blow off steam.

Every calorie counts.

Yes, You Can Still Have That Burger on Saturday

Good news: you can eat a cheeseburger if you want to! And drink a few beers, if that's your thing! You can eat whatever you want so long as you accept responsibility for it and factor it into the math.

You're an adult—at least I hope so.[56] As an adult, you decide what to eat and how much of it to eat. You need to own the decisions you make, especially when those decisions don't support your goals.

I'm sorry if this sounds like a tirade about personal responsibility. Maybe you were expecting me to say, *Go for it!* or *TREAT YO' SELF!* But the common approach to cheat meals is all wrong, because:

> **You don't cheat anyone when you eat food. You decide to eat it.**

You might enjoy eating something that isn't in line with the macro/deficit split you're aiming for, but you aren't getting ahead when you eat that stuff. You aren't gaming the system. You are sidestepping your goals, hopefully momentarily.

Banish the word "cheat" from your meal-planning approach right now. It's okay to enjoy an occasional meal that undermines your goals, but let's establish a different term for those meals. Here are alternate words to describe eating that burger on Saturday night: *splurging, indulging, treating yourself,* or maybe *slacking off.* When I eat something counterproductive to my goals, I call it an *off-plan* choice.

Examples:

My kid has a birthday party at a bowling alley this weekend, and they only sell hot dogs and fries, so I'll probably go *off-plan*.

Ben & Jerry's came out with a new flavor called "Better than Sex," so I'm going to have an *off-plan* treat tonight.

Screw it. I want this Big Mac. I'm going *off-plan*.

You might think this sounds like an inconsequential distinction, but it's not. Even when I go off-plan, **I still track my calories.** I don't "cheat." I own my off-plan decisions, and I acknowledge them even when they are mistakes.

For example, last weekend I went *crazy off-plan* at my in-laws' house. They had a massive tub of M&M's from Costco, and I kept hitting it like it was going out of style. I knew those M&M's undermined my goals, but I wanted them! I *decided* to eat them. I don't feel bad about that. I didn't cheat—I decided to eat something I wanted.

Did I track those calories? *You better bet I did.* Every last handful of M&M's went into MyFitnessPal. I owned my decision, and I don't feel guilty about eating those M&M's at all.

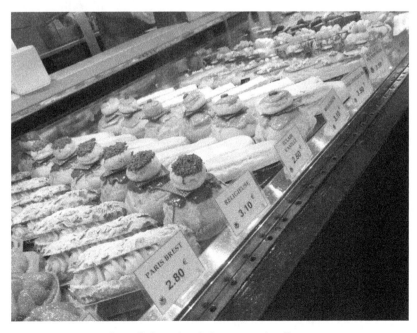

Some off-plan options during a recent trip to France.

Tracking calories—all of them, even and especially the off-plan ones—divorces you from compulsive eating. Compulsive eating makes us fat. Mindlessly snacking without intention makes us fat. Consciously deciding to eat something—taking responsibility for it—empowers us in our pursuit of improvement.

You can eat whatever you want, but you need to account for it in the context of your goals. **You need to own it,** *without feeling guilt or shame.* The science isn't judging you. The math continues to work regardless of your emotions. Don't feel guilty about those M&M's! These are *your* goals, and you are doing the best you can. Honor yourself by acknowledging the math, and you will feel better about the ~~mistakes~~ choices you make.

So, How Often Can You Go Off-Plan?

Only you can answer that question. What are your goals? How far do you have to go to reach them? And how do you feel at this moment, staring down that doughnut at your sister's wedding? Before you decide how often you want to eat something off-plan, ask yourself why you want to eat that thing in the first place: Do you like the taste of it? How does it affect your body? Are you eating it because it makes you feel a certain way?

FOOD AS A DRUG

Sometimes our bodies are out of sync. This can be physical, such as a cold or an injury, but it can also be emotional, due to stress. During moments of emotional duress we crave foods that make us feel better—"comfort foods." Many of us were trained from a young age to associate certain foods with an emotional state. Desserts for celebration, salty foods on game day, fried foods for relaxation, and so on. Then, in times of stress, we turn to these foods to recreate the celebratory feelings we've assigned to them. These learned behaviors formed habits that, for many of us, can be difficult to break.

However, some eating patterns stem from more than habits. Certain foods can and do alter your brain chemistry. For instance, a study at Princeton University found that sugar provokes a dopamine response in the brain that can be compared to morphine, cocaine, nicotine, and alcohol.[57] The dopamine response fosters dependencies similar to those of other addictive substances.

It's the hallmark of a chemical addiction. This differs from person to person based on your genetic predisposition to process certain foods.

Some doctors may disparage using the word "addiction" to describe compulsive sugar intake because the physiological effects aren't as devastating as opioid use, for instance.[58] They prefer to categorize food addictions as behavioral addictions, instead of chemical dependencies.

"Addiction" connotes many things. People say the word casually to describe the Netflix show they are *binge-watching*. People also use it to describe a devastating dependency on a substance or behavior. Maybe the word is too powerful to describe compulsive food cravings, but it's the word I use.

In my opinion, any substance that provokes the pleasure center of the brain has the potential to be addictive. Of course, this depends on the nature of the individual who consumes it, but these substances can be addictive even in the smallest amounts for some people. As such, I feel that it's irresponsible for any medical professional to claim that food addictions are not as dangerous as other drugs, alcohol, nicotine, etc. You need to ascertain how certain foods affect your mind, and then act accordingly.

Are You Addicted to Sugar?

Science has proven that sugar makes you "feel good" on a chemical level. That is indisputable. People don't enjoy sugar because of how it feels in the mouth, but because of the reaction it provokes in their brain. (Have you ever eaten a bowl of table sugar because you liked how it tasted?) Like any chemically addictive substance, sugar provokes a physiological response in your body—a *high*. Each individual handles that high differently. Some people enjoy it and then move on, while others develop a compulsion to seek it out again and again.

Manufacturers add sugar to products because of this reaction, and they've been steadily adding more and more sugar to their products for decades. A recent World Health Organization study quoted one food industry executive as saying there's been an "arms race for taste" among manufacturers.[59] As companies compete for customers, they've added more and more sugar to their products to beat out their competitors. But the race isn't merely to increase *sweetness*. Using sugar to make foods addictive so that you crave them is one of the ways manufacturers ensure the economic viability of their products in the marketplace. It's a function of the food-industrial complex—a system that prioritizes sales over the physical health of consumers.

Food manufacturers are like drug dealers. They aim to hook people on their products for profit. Coca-Cola used to have actual coca (cocaine) in it. Now it uses sugar to provide a similar "fix."

It's your choice whether you use the word "addiction" to describe the way sugar affects you. Either way, be conscious of how it alters your mood, and avoid consuming it mindlessly.

And please check the labels. Why do canned vegetables contain sugar? It's not a preservative, so ask yourself *why the hell is it in there?*

Which Foods Do You Crave?

Sugar is my monkey. I crave sugar in times of stress. When I am tired or upset, I want sugar. For other people it's fat, and for others it might be salt or something else. Whatever it is for you, make no mistake that some corporation has engineered junk food to satisfy that craving. They sell a product to make you *feel* better, and there is a high likelihood that you overindulge in that food when you feel off your game.

We're not robots. Sometimes our minds are out of whack, and eating for comfort is an easy solution. The thing you need to do is recognize that you are out of whack, and then decide *if* and *how far* you are willing to lean into that craving. If you crave something sweet and decide to eat it, try to have a plan in place for getting back on-plan. Look forward to reconnecting to your goals when you feel a little better.

Again, poor eating isn't a mistake; it's a decision. Decisions add up over time. What you decide to eat either helps or hinders your goals. Acknowledge your feelings and take responsibility for your choices. It's not cheating when you're aware of your reasons for making that choice, even if your reason is *comfort*.

REGULARLY SCHEDULED OFF-PLAN MEALS

I'm not a fan of regularly scheduled off-plan meals. Adding an extra 2,000 calories on weekends can erase whatever healthy deficit you've achieved during the week. (And the odds are that you won't make up for it with cardio, so don't get me started on that excuse.)

Why set yourself up for failure by planning to undo the hard work you did all week? Again, if you feel like you need a break on the weekends, that's your call to make. But do the math! Check your deficit and see what you gain or lose by scheduling yourself to go off-plan every weekend. If you're able to splurge on Saturdays while still maintaining a deficit for the week, then go for it. You track your calories even when you indulge, so you know exactly how much fat you expect to lose based on your deficit calculations.

But if you're one of those people who don't understand why they aren't losing weight, there's a fair chance that you're erasing your deficit by overeating on weekends.

Regular Special Occasions

What about a weekly "date night" or "friends' night out"? If you schedule an off-plan meal every weekend because you have a standing date night with your spouse or friends, I fully support that. If you enjoy hot dogs with your kids after Little League every Tuesday, that's wonderful. Those are valuable opportunities to socialize with people you love, and food can be a part of that. But track those hot dog calories and macros, and factor them into your meal planning for the week. Remember that all calories count. Balance your goals against your lifestyle and obligations.

Don't Plan a Splurge Without a Reason

If you schedule a splurge each week because you feel the need to eat something bad to feel good, then you should speak with a therapist. I'm serious. If you spend the week in diet purgatory—waiting it out until the weekend when you will eat whatever you want—then you should talk to a professional. If you eat junk food as a reward because you think of your other meals as punishment, you may have an eating disorder or an addiction that requires professional attention.

Eating disorders are serious. They require personal guidance well beyond the scope of this book. If you schedule binges or succumb to compulsive eating, please seek medical advice. There's no shame in asking for help.

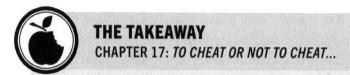

THE TAKEAWAY
CHAPTER 17: *TO CHEAT OR NOT TO CHEAT...*

If you eat something unhealthy, don't think of it as a "cheat" meal. Think of it as a calculated decision, and always consider how each choice you make factors into the bigger picture. *(Small goals, remember?)*

I prefer to say *off-plan*, which acknowledges that I have a plan but I'm temporarily taking a break from it.

The key to eating off-plan is to think about what you are eating before you eat it. More specifically, consider why you are eating it.

> » Are you eating this thing because you are stressed?

> » Are you eating this thing because it's a social celebration?

> » Are you eating this thing because you enjoy the taste or you want to try something new?

> » Are you eating this thing because it provokes a chemical response in your body and you crave that response?

Don't ignore your goals. It's okay to go off-plan as long as you remain mindful of your choices. Going off-plan does not mean losing track of your goals and the bigger picture. Don't try to "cheat." You will lose.

Maintain focus on your overall objective: to get the body of your dreams.

> » If you are okay with how that off-plan treat impacts your weekly deficit, go for it. But be conscious of your decisions.

> » Only you can decide if you are reaching for that fifth slice of pizza because you want it, or because you are bored.

This isn't hard. You know how much to eat in order to reach your goals. You know the math. But you also know that you aren't perfect and that life gets in the way. Do your best to plan, including the times you anticipate going off-plan, and **don't forget to track every single decision along the way.**

PART THREE

STRENGTH TRAINING

STRENGTH TRAINING IS YOUR BEST WEAPON

I do it as a therapy. I do it as something to keep me alive. We all need a little discipline. Exercise is my discipline.

JACK LALANNE

WHAT IS STRENGTH TRAINING?

Props to whomever wrote the current Wikipedia description, which reads:

> *Strength training is a type of physical exercise specializing in the use of resistance to induce muscular contraction, which builds the strength, anaerobic endurance, and size of skeletal muscles.*

Typical strength-training programs require you to lift weights in repetition, creating resistance against a muscle or muscle group in a controlled sequence. You quantify, qualify, and record the data from each repetition to track improvements.

While there are many new methods for creating resistance against our muscles—like flipping tires in a parking lot—I use the terms "strength training," "weight training," and "weightlifting" interchangeably.

When I say strength training, I'm talking about <u>weightlifting</u>. It's typically done in a gym, with barbells, dumbbells, machines, bands, and body weight.

Maybe your preferred method of creating resistance against muscular contraction involves something other than traditional weights. If so, I assume that the resistance you use is as reliably quantifiable as, say, seeing the "25 lb" sticker on a dumbbell. If the amount of weight you move is not *explicit*, you aren't strength training.

The first thing to know about strength training is this:

**Strength training is the only way to
get a lean, muscular physique.**

That's a bold statement, and it also assumes the following:

- You *want* a lean, muscular physique.

- You *don't want* to look soft, skinny-fat, or as skinny as possible.*

- You *want* to be healthy.

- You *are not* an aspiring endurance athlete who requires a specific body type to compete in a particular sport.

If you disagree with any of these statements, then you can ignore my advice and skip the rest of this book. However, since you've read this far I assume you are interested in achieving these goals. You'd like to be balanced, athletic, and healthy. You want your body to work efficiently, and you want your clothes to fit. You might have higher aspirations for muscle growth—maybe you want to be a professional bodybuilder—but you're probably not ready to think about that yet.

So, how does strength training factor into achieving these goals?

STRENGTH TRAINING BENEFITS

You need to strength train as part of any serious exercise program. Let's break down the benefits of regular strength training, and how it impacts your goals.

---

* Please don't try to disappear. We need you here.

Muscle Burns More Calories Than Fat

Muscle mass requires more metabolic activity during rest, meaning that the more muscle you have, the more calories you burn just by breathing. That means your BMR (and therefore your TDEE) increases in conjunction with an increase in muscle mass. A person with more muscle mass burns more calories than another person with less muscle mass, just by being alive.

According to Christopher Wharton, a doctor, personal trainer, and researcher with the Rudd Center for Food Policy and Obesity at Yale University:

> **Ten pounds of muscle at rest burns 50 calories in a day, while 10 pounds of fat only burns 20 calories in a day.**[60]

How does that math work in real life? Let's use my original DEXA scan figures as an example. I was 5'10", 178 pounds with 27% body fat and six pounds of bone. I had the following body composition (rounded for ease of discussion): **47 lb of fat and 125 lb of lean tissue.**

We'll assume the lean mass is 100% muscle for the sake of this equation. Using Dr. Wharton's research, my fat and muscle tissue burned a total of 719 calories at rest each day.

$$[(47 \text{ lb}/10) \times 20 \text{ cal}] + [(125 \text{ lb}/10) \times 50 \text{ cal}] = \textbf{719 calories}$$

But what would happen if I replaced 10 pounds of fat with 10 pounds of muscle?

$$[((47 \text{ lb} - 10 \text{ lb})/10) \times 20 \text{ cal}] + [((125 \text{ lb} + 10 \text{ lb})/10) \times 50 \text{ cal}]$$
$$= \textbf{749 calories}$$

That's a difference of 40 calories per day *at rest*. That means I wouldn't have to lift a finger to burn that extra 40 calories. That might not seem significant, but over time it makes a huge difference:

40 x 7 days = 280 extra calories burned at rest per week
280 calories x 4 weeks = 1,120 extra calories burned at rest per month
1,120 x 3 = **3,360 extra calories burned at rest in 3 months**

That figure, 3,360 calories, is almost a pound of fat burned in three months without any exercise. **That's like losing four pounds per year just by being**

alive. That's why people with more muscle mass are often leaner, too. Their bodies burn more calories at rest, and this burn increases exponentially with exercise.

Using my DEXA scans as an example, note the increase in BMR between my first and second scans:

- At the time of my first DEXA scan, I weighed 178 lb: 48 lb of fat, 124 lb of lean tissue, and 6 lb of bone. **My BMR was 1,578 calories/day**.
- At the time of my second DEXA scan, I weighed 158 lb: 22 lb of fat and 136 lb of lean tissue. **My BMR jumped up to 1,684 calories/day**.

I weighed 13 pounds less at the time of my second scan, but my body required 106 more calories each day as a minimum. That's an extra 106 calories burned each day with no extra effort at all. I need more calories every day, even though I weigh less. The additional muscle I gained requires more calories than the fat I previously carried.

An extra 106 calories a day might not seem like many calories to you, but it adds up fast: 106 calories burned per day x 365 days = 38,690 calories burned in a year. **That's the equivalent of burning 11 pounds of fat**.

Can you visualize what losing 11 pounds of fat would look like on you?

The most compelling reason to strength train is that more muscle mass makes it easier for you to create a caloric deficit.

Strength Training Improves the Body's Ability to Metabolize Sugars Effectively

Muscle mass is designed to pull glucose from the bloodstream and deliver it to muscle cells. An increase in muscle mass means more glucose is removed from the bloodstream, thereby lowering blood sugar levels. Strength training equips your body to process glucose more efficiently in the long term. Your system uses carbohydrates more effectively and becomes less likely to store simple sugars as fat. That's another way strength training promotes sustained, long-term fat loss.

This underscores my suggestion that simple carbohydrates are best consumed in coordination with your workouts. By consuming simple carbohydrates in coordination with strength training, you supply your body with the tools it needs to build muscle in response to muscle fatigue.

Strength Training Increases Positive Body Image, Regardless of Actual Aesthetic Improvements

When you lift weights, you feel better about how you look, regardless of how you actually look. A 2005 study found that changes in perceived muscularity and body composition were significantly associated with changes in body satisfaction, irrespective of physical changes in those areas. The research indicates that perceived improvements to your level of fitness have a more significant impact on body image than actual increases in strength and size, or decreases in body fat.[61] Likewise, a 2015 study indicated "significant improvements" in body image among older women after a 10-week, twice-weekly strength training program.[62]

Training improves your self-image even if the tangible results aren't objectively quantifiable. *Why?* It's probably a combination of both the physical and mental changes that happen in conjunction with regular strength training. The physical improvements are guaranteed, even if they aren't immediately noticeable:

- Increased strength
- Increased mobility and better posture
- Increased physical stamina
- Improved cardiovascular health
- Increased bone density

However, the improvements to your mental health are even more valuable than these physical changes. Strength training has been shown to decrease anxiety and depression,[63] in part due to the endorphins released during exercise, but also by improving sleep and exposing your mind to repeated physical stress.[64] It also improves your mood and attitude by providing "an opportunity to overcome obstacles in a controlled, predictable environment."[65]

Strength training creates a simple opportunity to accomplish a set of short-term goals in a controlled environment. The sense of accomplishment you feel when you achieve these goals increases self-perception and confidence. This confidence encourages you to aim for *even bigger* goals! Then the cycle repeats.

**When you lift weights, your confidence
increases, which makes it easier to achieve other
goals, including your daily caloric deficit.**

Regular strength training improves your self-image by making you feel successful. The sense of achievement you feel after working out kills your cravings for comfort foods because you already feel great.

Also, strength training has been proven to decrease stress. That's vital to any fat-loss plan because your body's stress response mimics the starvation response. When you are stressed, your body stifles nonessential functions to conserve energy in case of an emergency. However, stress differs from actual starvation because it originates in your mind, often in conjunction with a sense of *powerlessness*.

Conversely, when you lift weights, you repeatedly exert control over a straightforward situation: moving a dumbbell. Lifting weights reassures your brain that you have control of the situation on a subconscious level, by relieving mental stress. It makes you feel powerful! You are voluntarily pushing these weights around, so your mind assumes there is no emergency, and therefore no need to conserve energy.

Ninety-nine percent of my stress originates in scenarios when I feel powerless in some way. My time in the gym makes me feel like I have more control over my life. I'm working toward easily verifiable goals, like increasing the weight I lift or squeezing out one more rep. An extra set of biceps curls doesn't guarantee I'm the master of *everything* in my life, but it does assure me that *I've mastered something at this moment*. That feeling of accomplishment trickles into everything else I do for the rest of the day.

Strength training strengthens your mind and mood. Good mental health makes it easier to achieve your fat-loss goals and anything else you want to achieve. When you feel confident, the sky is the limit!

The Problem With Being "Skinny-Fat"

I don't know how else to say this. You don't want to be *skinny-fat*. For those who are unfamiliar with this term, it's used to describe someone thin who isn't truly fit or muscular. It's not just an aesthetic distinction; it's medically proven that it's unhealthy to be skinny-fat.

By my definition, a "skinny-fat" person doesn't exercise but stays thin because they are malnourished. It's the look of a person who eats ramen noodles for dinner, smokes too much weed (or worse, cigarettes), and gets their carbohydrates from beer and potato chips.

It's my understanding that skinny-fat people often store excess visceral fat without realizing it. Visceral fat surrounds your organs, and it's a precursor to many serious health concerns.

Squeezing into pants with a 29-inch waist *does not* ensure you're healthy. The skinny-fat person might be camouflaging critical health concerns, like prediabetes, heart disease, or cancer. A high body fat percentage on a thin frame is still dangerous, especially if the individual is unaware of it.

Conversely, strength training creates metabolic health from the inside out. A regular strength-training program tunes your body for metabolic performance, improves circulation and cardiovascular health, and helps prevent some of the health concerns above.

I'm not talking about getting bigger muscles; you can still be thin and have excellent physical and mental health. You don't need massive muscles to be healthy! But developing your muscles through regular strength training increases your health no matter your size.

STRENGTH TRAINING MYTHS

I want to address some common misconceptions about strength training in case you still aren't convinced by the benefits. Let's dispel the myths people use as excuses to avoid lifting weights.

MYTH NUMBER 1:

Lifting weights will make me look like a bodybuilder. I don't want to look like that!

FALSE! If everyone were capable of looking like a bodybuilder with regular strength training, there would be a lot more gigantic guys in the gym. I've never worked out at a gym where there were more than one or two people with a bodybuilder physique working out at any given time.

Gaining that kind of muscle demands way more time and effort in the gym than the average person requires to get to their next level of fitness. You can't automatically become a bodybuilder with regular strength training.

MYTH NUMBER 2:

*I want a more muscular body, but the only way to
make that happen is with steroids, so why even try
to do it naturally?*

FALSE! Have you seen the statue of David? Would David's body qualify as muscular? Do you think the bodies Michelangelo sketched as a study for David were using steroids? Of course not!

Germans invented synthesized testosterone (steroids) in 1935.[66] That's right—Nazis created steroids... way after David.

History is full of muscular people who never used steroids. You do not need to use steroids to achieve a lean, muscular physique.

MYTH NUMBER 3:

*Strength training is expensive. I can't afford a
fancy gym or a personal trainer.*

WRONG AGAIN! Like steroids, commercial gyms with fitness machines are a relatively new invention. People were getting fit before gyms or personal trainers became a thing.

Yes, you'll benefit from a gym with essential weight-training equipment (mostly free weights). Gym memberships are relatively cheap now, and the program I follow utilizes standard equipment found in most gyms. But a gym membership isn't mandatory. You can strength train effectively with bags of sand as long as you know the weight of each bag. Where there's a will, there's a way! Strength training is all about adding quantifiable resistance against your muscles. You don't need anything *fancy* for that.

MYTH NUMBER 4:

I don't have time to strength train. I'm too busy!

BULLSHIT! You can transform your body with an hour in the gym three to five times each week. That's a minimal investment of time to reach your fitness goals.

I'm super busy, too. I have a family and lots of other work to do. (No, writing this book is not my full-time job.) **If I can make it to the gym four or five times a week, so can you.**

FINAL THOUGHT

These are just some of the reasons I believe you need strength training to achieve meaningful, sustained fat loss. I'll compare strength training (anaerobic exercise) to cardiovascular (aerobic) exercise in a subsequent chapter. There are benefits to doing cardio, but later we will examine why cardio on its own is *not* an effective way to train.

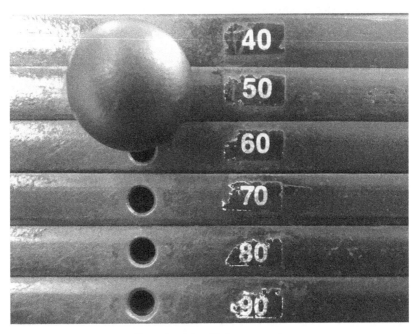

Strength training. It's time to get on it.

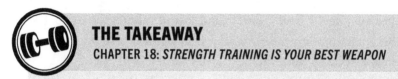

THE TAKEAWAY
CHAPTER 18: *STRENGTH TRAINING IS YOUR BEST WEAPON*

If you want to be lean and muscular, strength training is essential to reaching your goals.

Muscle mass burns more calories than fat mass. These calories add up and ultimately make a huge difference in your total caloric deficit.

Regular strength training (and an increase in muscle mass) improves your body's ability to metabolize sugars efficiently. The more muscle mass you carry, the less likely you are to store excess sugars as fat.

Regular strength training improves your body image regardless of actual aesthetic changes. An increase in positive body image means more confidence and better mental preparation to achieve your goals.

Strength training decreases stress, which also makes it easier for you to pursue goals.

An increase in muscle mass has countless physiological benefits. Losing fat without simultaneously developing your muscles (the "skinny-fat" syndrome) can mask health problems with an otherwise thin physique.

Bottom line: if you're not strength training, you're missing a vital part of the fat-loss equation. **Get on it!**

CHAPTER 19

HOW TO TRACK YOUR GAINS

In God we trust. All others must bring data.

ANONYMOUS

DATA RULES

You already know that tracking your calories is the only reliable way to lose fat. You have a system for tracking changes in your body fat percentage, and you're probably taking progress pics to hold yourself accountable, too. This data reveals which calculations are working and which might need to be tweaked. Data from our small, daily goals keeps us excited, responsible, and in control of our trajectory.

It's essential to track our strength-training progress for these same reasons. When you train, you're sure to notice positive changes to the way you look and feel. Tracking numerical data about your workouts helps you quantify these changes without the subjective filter of your ego clouding the truth.

For example, you may have gained an inch in your biceps, but you might not casually notice that in the mirror because you're stressed about something else. By maintaining an accurate record of your improvements, you have factual data to refer to whenever you question your results, regardless of your frame of mind.

Tracking this data helps you to qualify your strengths and weaknesses *objectively*. Numbers don't lie. If you aren't happy with the gains you're making in a particular muscle group, you might decide to prioritize that muscle next month.

Data rules. If you're new to weightlifting and you need help starting to collect data, you can use the following metrics to chart your progress in the gym, the same way you track your calories.

METRICS FOR TRACKING STRENGTH-TRAINING GAINS

Remember, for our purposes, *strength training* is synonymous with *weight training*. If you want to lose fat, you should be lifting weights—preferably in a gym—several days a week. It's essential that:

- The weight is **measured** (i.e., you know how much it weighs); and

- The motion is **repeated**, which creates a multiplier for that amount of weight because you are moving it a certain number of times during a defined duration.

These factors provide you with two ideal data points to track:

Total volume: the amount of weight you move multiplied by the number of times you move it.

Total time under tension: the amount of time a muscle works against the resistance you've placed in front of it (i.e., how long it endures the stress).

Use a notebook or, easier yet, a smartphone app to track these metrics. I've been using the Strong app on iOS for several years now, and I can't imagine working out without it. (Check it out at www.strong.app.) It provides real-time data for my reps in comparison to previous workouts and builds terrific charts and graphs to show my progress.

The following sections explain why I believe total volume and total time under tension are the two most viable data points to consider when evaluating your progress in the gym.

TOTAL VOLUME

The total combined amount of weight you can lift in all sets of an exercise is the most notable indication of your improvement. Total volume is a complete sum of the weight you moved for each repetition of an exercise, multiplied by the number of reps, multiplied by the number of sets. In other words, it's *all of the weight for an exercise represented as one large number.*

Total Volume = Weight x Reps x Sets

Here's an example of a total volume calculation using a session of squats I performed in a recent workout:

Set #1: 155 lb x 12 reps = 1,860 lb
Sets #2 & #3: 135 lb x 15 reps x 2 sets = 4,050 lb
Set #4: 155 lb x 8 reps = 1,240 lb

Total volume: 7,150 lb

That is an enormous number! I like tracking enormous numbers because they give me a bird's-eye view of the data. Any extraneous variables are marginalized throughout several sets, and any reps with poor form are also absorbed into the average. What do I mean by that? We can't *always* have perfect form. There will be bad reps we don't notice. By tracking total weight for an exercise, the weight we lifted during any *less-than-perfect* reps gets averaged in with the reps we executed correctly.

Once you know your total volume for an exercise, you track it against previous workouts. Tracking total volume makes it easy to review gains because small increases in weight are clearer in aggregate.

In the example above, I increased the weight on the bar for my last set by five pounds (a 2.5-pound weight on each side). That seems like a tiny amount, but over eight reps it increased my total volume for this exercise from 7,110 pounds to 7,150 pounds. I can appreciate that increase, even though the actual amount of weight I added was pretty small. Seeing that I increased the total weight by 40 pounds resonates more than seeing I only added a 2.5-pound plate to each side of the bar.

Additionally, tracking the total volume also values an increase in reps. If I maintain the same weight on the bar during this week's session, but I squeak out an extra rep, that increase in total weight factors into the metric I track. As a result, the increase in reps impacts the metric I'm following the same way an increase in weight would.

Those are the reasons why I track my workouts with one big number: *the total volume I've lifted during each exercise.*

Tracking Total Volume Is Simple

If you track with an app, the app should add up the total weight for you on the fly, presenting the increase in total volume for that exercise after each set. Useful workout apps also calculate and chart changes in total volume week-over-week, making it easy to see improvements.

If you use a paper notebook in the gym—*ain't nothing wrong with that!*—then I suggest summing the total volume of weight after each set during rests. You could do it after your workout, but then you're waiting to review the data instead of pushing yourself during the current workout.

TOTAL TIME UNDER TENSION

The second primary data point you might consider tracking is time under tension, a.k.a. *TUT*. Again, this is the total amount of time—in minutes and seconds—that my muscles fight against resistance.

It's not as easy to track this number day-to-day, so I don't, but I reflect on it continuously while lifting. I think about it in two ways during my workouts:

- I think about (and adjust) the tempo and **rhythm** of my exercises; and

- I consider how minimizing or maximizing the amount of time I spend resting between sets affects my **time under tension.**

Rhythm

How does rhythm, or tempo, impact time under tension? A slower rhythm means greater time under tension.

Example: If I lower the weight in a controlled rhythm, I maintain tension on the muscle for the second half of the rep, thereby *increasing* my TUT. However, if I drop the weight on the return, I cut short the potential time under tension (i.e., I *decrease* TUT).

Even though I don't actively track tempo, I *consider* it during each rep. Maintaining a consistent rhythm ensures that I focus on the negative portion of the rep, a.k.a. the eccentric movement, a.k.a. the return to starting position.

Making the most out of the negative portion of a rep helps stress the muscle by increasing time under tension.

If you decide to track TUT, one way to improve your set might be to increase the amount of time you spend on each motion in the rep week-over-week. For example, if you took three seconds to curl your biceps during each rep this week, you might try to increase that time to four seconds next week. That would be an increase in time under tension.

Regardless of your tempo, never let a weight "drop" or "snap back" on the return motion. It's dangerous, and you cheat your muscles out of half of the exercise. Maintaining a steady rhythm forces you to consider your time under tension and to maximize it in each repetition. The amount of time your muscle can remain under tension indicates your level of strength, and it's worth considering this factor even if you don't actively record the data.

Even without tracking TUT as a metric for gauging improvement, you should factor it into determining the quality of your workouts. (I write about the benefits of tempo training in an upcoming chapter.)

THE "ONE-REP MAX"

A third metric some people track is the *one-rep maximum*. Your one-rep maximum indicates the heaviest amount of weight you can perform for a single rep. One-rep maxes can be fun to consider, but they aren't a reliable benchmark for tracking progress. Myriad factors influence this data because there are lots of things that may help or hinder you when you push, pull, or lift something heavy just one time:

- You might be angry or desperate, and therefore naturally amped up.

- You could be *chemically* amped because your coffee just kicked in.

- You might feel extra confident because you are competing or showing off for a friend.

- Your glucose levels or the amount of energy you have stored in this exact moment might be higher than yesterday because you ate something different.

There are formulas for tracking a one-rep max based on total volume, and some workout apps do it for you automatically. It's amusing to look at that number casually, but it isn't a reliable indication of improvement either. Even though it is based on your total volume, it means averaging that number... which makes it *inaccurate* as a measurement of your one-rep max. A one-rep max is the weight you can lift one time; it's *not* an average of the weight you lifted during a set which may have included complicated rhythms, varying rest periods, and general fatigue.

Skip tracking your one-rep max unless there is a specific reason you need to know how much weight you can lift in a single rep. *Like, if you're headed to the Olympics or something.*

Tracking changes in total volume or total time under tension yields a reliable data set to help you quantify your gains. Understanding this data and applying that knowledge to your workouts makes it easy to set new small goals during every workout. That's the difference between making gains and... *whatever that guy is doing over there with the cable. He's kinda flailing his arms around really fast.* Don't be that guy.

THE TAKEAWAY
CHAPTER 19: *HOW TO TRACK YOUR GAINS*

You need to track data from your strength-training workouts to ensure that what you're doing in the gym actually works.

Tracking your gains keeps you motivated, identifies weak spots, and helps you set small goals for every workout. It keeps you accountable for the decisions you make. Hard data is more reliable than looking in a mirror because numbers don't change with emotions or good lighting.

There are two primary indicators of strength to track during workouts: the **total volume** of weight lifted and the **total time under tension**.

» Total volume is the sum of all the weight you've lifted during an exercise. It's the amount of weight on the bar multiplied by the number of reps in the set multiplied by the number of sets. Total volume is the most reliable, straightforward, and encouraging metric to track your progress in the gym.

» Total time under tension, or **TUT**, is the amount of time in minutes and seconds that your muscles are under tension. It's challenging to track TUT as a means of comparing your progress from week to week, but you should reflect on it during your sets and reps. Aim for consistent increases in time under tension even though you probably won't record those numbers.

The eccentric (i.e., negative) movement in a rep—when you return the weight to its starting point—counts toward total time under tension. If you drop the weight back to the starting point, you short your potential time under tension for that rep.

I don't recommend using your one-rep maximum to chart improvement. This number is wildly inaccurate because it's influenced by myriad factors. It's fun to consider your one-rep max, but don't base any serious strength-training program around improving it.

COMPOUND EXERCISES vs. ISOLATION EXERCISES

Squat like your ass depends on it. Because it does.

UNKNOWN

HOW TO CHOOSE YOUR EXERCISES

Now you know that strength training is essential to getting the body you want. Perhaps you're thinking, "Which exercises should I do? What am I doing in this gym? And what about CrossFit?!"

Calm down. Take a breath, and don't be overwhelmed by the endless supply of weight-training plans available on the Internet. You need to start with a simple program comprised of a few conventional exercises, especially if you're trying to lean out. It's less complicated than you expect.

There are essentially two kinds of exercises: *compound exercises* and *isolation exercises.*

Compound exercises require more than one joint, and multiple muscle groups working in conjunction to perform a movement.

Isolation exercises entail a single joint and emphasize a single primary muscle group.

Your training plan should feature a combination of these two types of exercises. Let's examine the broad benefits of each category so that you are equipped to choose the right exercise for the job.

COMPOUND EXERCISES

Compound exercises engage multiple muscle groups and joints, and they mimic the compound movements we use in real-world situations. Compound exercises are the cornerstone of my training because they increase practical strength, they allow for a greater total volume of resistance, and they improve balance and coordination.

Practical strength is the strength needed for everyday movements you do outside the gym. When was the last time you decided to lift a piece of furniture using only your biceps? *Probably never.* That's because it's easier and safer to lift heavy objects with multiple muscle groups, instead of limiting the work to a single muscle. Coordinating the movements between several muscles and spreading the stress across multiple joints provides more power and greater stability during the movement. Compound exercises increase your strength, efficiency, and aptitude for performing similar movements in real-world applications.

Compound exercises also allow you to train with greater total volume because they engage more muscle mass. More mass means more power, which in turn means heavier weight. Training with higher volume leads to greater gains in size and strength.[67] In lieu of increasing volume by increasing the number of sets you use to engage a specific muscle group, compound exercises allow for higher volume *per set* because you can naturally lift more weight when using multiple muscle groups. Although that higher total volume is spread across different muscles, the distribution of force is determined by your specific anatomy. Compound exercises utilize a distribution of force that mimics the way your muscles coordinate power naturally based on your frame. That in turn leads to a balanced musculature, instead of some muscles being disproportionately larger or smaller than others. Compound exercises build muscle in symmetry with the shape of your body.

Compound exercises also increase the resilience of connective tissues because they force your body to coordinate the *secondary* parts of the mechanisms required to perform the motion. These include bones, ligaments, and tendons. You engage these tissues during compound lifts in ways similar to how you engage them in the practical movements, which improves their strength and stability in daily life.

Additionally, compound exercises improve balance because they require full-body coordination. There are multiple motions involved in a compound movement; even when compound exercises appear to be a single motion, they require several actions, by definition. And you also engage your core muscles for additional stabilization. Coordinating all of these muscles and joints improves your balance in real-world applications.

For these reasons, I make compound exercises the foundation of my training program, and I suggest that you do as well. Begin each workout with compound exercises, and strive to make incremental increases in total volume, week-over-week.

ISOLATION EXERCISES

Isolation exercises do just that: they *isolate* a single major muscle group.* The movement requires only *one* joint to engage, and it aims to strengthen the contraction in *one* muscle group.

Some people argue that isolation exercises don't really exist, because all exercises require ancillary or peripheral muscle and joint engagement in some way. That's true, if you want to be technical. But my definition of an isolation exercise is one that is intended to isolate a single muscle. How much you engage other muscles or joints to perform the movement will depend on your skill level, the amount of weight you choose, and your genetics. However, your goal remains the same regardless of these factors: *to isolate a single muscle group.* I suggest incorporating isolation exercises at the end of your workout in order to minimize these variables, so you can really focus on isolating your intended target.

Isolation exercises are great when you want to completely exhaust a specific muscle. I like to think of isolation exercises as the icing on the cake. *Mmm, dessert metaphor.* These exercises require less weight to reach muscle fatigue, because they engage less muscle mass. Capitalizing on this idea by programming isolation exercises at the end of your workout will likely improve your form, help you correct muscle imbalances, and protect your joints from catastrophic injury.

First, if you begin a workout with compound movements your muscles are already tired by the time you get to the isolation exercises. That means you have to use *even less weight* to train them to the point of total exhaustion. For example, I often perform biceps curls (a classic isolation exercise) with 10- or 12-pound dumbbells. That's not a substantial amount of weight. But

---

* Isolation exercises *may* require limited engagement of secondary muscle groups, but I qualify these exercises as being explicitly intended to train a single primary muscle group.

if I were to begin my workout with biceps curls, I'd have more energy so I might be tempted to grab a 40-pound dumbbell in each hand. I'd squeak out a set, and then my form would go to hell on the next one as that amount of weight became more challenging. I'd unconsciously begin to swing the dumbbells in subsequent sets, using momentum, or the muscles in my back, to move the dumbbells. This extraneous power is a substitute for the added power I could rely on during a compound movement. But none of the extra power from swinging the weight helps me to isolate my biceps! It defeats the entire purpose of the biceps curl.

However, if I've already performed compound exercises that incorporated my biceps, then I can *exhaust* them with much less weight. Less weight means it's easier for me to perform the exercise with the utmost precision. I can concentrate intently on the fundamental motion of the biceps curl: contracting my biceps *and nothing else*. I perform the exercise slowly and methodically, to ensure that I create tension in the specific muscle I'm targeting, instead of just trying to move a heavy weight.

Isolating a muscle lets you correct imbalances that may happen naturally based on your genetics, or as a result of other factors. You may notice that your biceps are underdeveloped in proportion to the rest of your arms. You can address that imbalance by adding isolation exercises to the end of your workout *after* you've already engaged your biceps in conjunction with complementary muscle groups. This is an opportunity to give them the extra push they need to grow, without re-prioritizing the way your muscles coordinate naturally. For example, biceps curls give my biceps a chance to make up for any weakness they exhibited during the round of pull-ups I did earlier in the workout.

Additionally, using less weight during isolation exercises is also safer because it means loading less resistance on a single joint. Consolidating pressure on one joint increases the risk of injury to that joint. The heavier the weight I lift, the more likely I am to jeopardize that joint. And there are lots of reasons a joint might be predisposed to injury, including previous injuries, joint dysfunction caused by a genetic predisposition, tendinitis, circulatory problems, arthritis, and more.

For example, I have several "slack" joints that are prone to slipping out. If I use less weight during isolation exercises I minimize the danger of injury if a particular joint slips. Joint failure under a 10-pound dumbbell will be less catastrophic than joint failure under a 40-pound dumbbell.

These are just some of the benefits of performing isolation exercises at the end of your workout routine, after compound exercises. However, you may see people at your gym choosing isolation exercises more often than compound exercises, or skipping compound movements altogether. *Why?*

One reason people prioritize isolation exercises is because they like to pump their *vanity muscles*. Vanity muscles for men are most commonly the chest, biceps, and shoulders. For women, they might be the booty, thighs, and tight abs. People emphasize these muscles with isolation exercises so they can flex, pose, and *take great Insta pics, brah!* They treat these as the most important muscles in the body, but they are not.

All of your muscles are important. *All* of your muscles have a purpose. You need to train *all* of them to create a proportionate, healthy physique and to avoid injuries. Don't skimp on a comprehensive training plan to make sure your arms look big for the club.

Use Machines Sparingly

Most weightlifting machines are intended for isolation exercises. That's because the pulley or arm of the machine can only move on a single axis, with a limited range of motion. These machines restrict the movement of other muscle groups, as well as bones and sometimes joints, with pads and benches.

Some people prefer to work out with machines because they appear simpler than compound movements. People seem to be less afraid of them. Restricting movement with comfy padding lessens the assumed risk of injury. Lots of people are intimidated by free weights, so they opt for machines.

But if you're serious about building a lean, muscular physique, you should limit your reliance on machines. Instead, learn to perform the primary compound exercises safely, with proper form. Use machines sparingly in conjunction with other isolation exercises *after* you've worked compound lifts, even if the machine was designed to mimic a compound movement.

Recent research supports the theory that free-weight exercises have a more significant physiological impact than similar exercises performed with machines. A study at the University of North Texas showed that lifters produced more testosterone and growth hormone after a series of squats than they did after using a leg press machine.[68]

Why do exercises with free weights cause the body to produce more testosterone and growth hormone? It might be because these exercises mimic the way your body has evolved to move, including related stresses throughout the body. A squat forces you to control the weight independently, during several positions. Conversely, a leg press machine restricts your range of motion and isolates your hips and upper body—something that would never happen in real life.

Your body is designed to push and pull using combinations of muscle groups and joints, not to perform a repetition with a perfect 90-degree angle. The increase in hormone production from compound exercises could be our bodies reacting predictably—with more hormones in response to tension—when performing movements that require more concentration, balance, and control of ancillary muscles and joints.

Most compound exercises require the use of free weights, while most machine exercises work to isolate parts of the body. This is yet another reason I prioritize compound lifts over isolation exercises.

PRIMARY EXERCISES

Here's a list of the exercises I consider to be essential to any foundational training program, separated by type. This list is by no means exhaustive, but it provides a sound framework for your weight-training program. (I've included a larger list of my preferred exercises at the back of the book, grouped by exercise type and muscle group.) The plans I've included at the back of the book also indicate a few additional exercises, but the following list is what I consider to be the *greatest hits*. You can create a rock-solid program with just these exercises.

Many of these exercises have multiple variations, each one targeting the muscles from a different angle. However, the standard form of each exercise listed here is all you really need when you're starting out. Most of us could spend a lifetime trying to master the form of these standards. Together they incorporate all the movements needed to train every major muscle group in your body.

There are many websites and YouTube videos you can reference if you're unfamiliar with an exercise, and I encourage you to check them out. Even better, hire a personal trainer to help you develop proper form. Working with a qualified professional will put you on a path toward mastery. You won't need to pay a trainer forever, but proper instruction at the beginning can set you up for a lifetime of success... no matter your current age.

PRIMARY COMPOUND EXERCISES

Squat	*Hamstrings, Quads, Glutes, Calves*
Bench Press	*Chest, Triceps, Shoulders*
Dips	*Chest, Triceps, Shoulders*
Standard Deadlift	*Upper & Lower Back, Glutes, Hamstrings*
Pull-ups	*Upper Back, Biceps, Forearms*
Barbell Rows	*Upper & Lower Back, Biceps*
Barbell Overhead Press	*Shoulders, Upper Back, Triceps, Chest*
Crunches (most variations)	*Abdominals*

PRIMARY ISOLATION EXERCISES

Leg Extension	*Quads*
Leg Curl	*Hamstrings*
Hip Thrusters	*Glutes*
Calf Raises	*Calves*
Biceps Curl	*Biceps*
Triceps Extension	*Triceps*
Lateral Raise	*Shoulders*
Lower Back Extension	*Lower Back*

Note: It's possible to perform many compound exercises in a "semi-isolated" mode by holding a dumbbell in each hand. However, I prefer to use barbells for compound exercises in most instances.

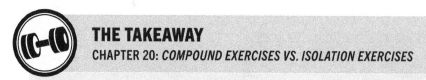

THE TAKEAWAY
CHAPTER 20: *COMPOUND EXERCISES VS. ISOLATION EXERCISES*

Most exercises can be categorized into one of two groups, compound exercises and isolation exercises:

» **Compound exercises** require more than one joint and multiple muscle groups working together to perform a movement.

» **Isolation exercises** focus on the movement of a single joint and a single primary muscle group.

Compound exercises mimic real-world movements. They allow you to move heavier weights because they incorporate more muscle mass. They are known to **increase practical strength for real-world applications, increase testosterone and growth hormone production, strengthen connective tissues, and improve balance.**

» Make compound exercises the foundation of your training program. Begin each workout with compound exercises and work toward incremental increases in volume each week.

Isolation exercises are great for leading a muscle group to exhaustion safely. Add them toward the end of your workout *after* your muscles are already fatigued by compound movements. That way, you require less weight to exhaust the muscle, which means placing less strain on a single joint. Using less weight decreases the potential for injury.

A list of exercises I recommend can be found at the end of the book.

» Prioritize compound movements in order to achieve muscular growth that complements your natural frame.

» Incorporate isolation exercises to completely fatigue specific muscles safely in order to address imbalances and weak spots.

» Programming your training in this order builds functional fitness, encourages a proportionate physique, and provides you with the most bang for your buck.

CHAPTER 21

STRENGTH, HYPERTROPHY, OR ENDURANCE?

Man often becomes what he believes himself to be. If I keep on saying to myself that I cannot do a certain thing, it is possible that I may end by really becoming incapable of doing it. On the contrary, if I have the belief that I can do it, I shall surely acquire the capacity to do it even if I may not have it at the beginning.

MAHATMA GANDHI

THREE APPROACHES TO TRAINING

I call it strength training, but gaining strength is only *one* potential benefit to lifting heavy weights. Weight training can yield three distinct effects:

- Increased **strength;**
- Increased **hypertrophy** (i.e., size); and
- Increased **endurance.**

When you first start training, you will probably increase strength in combination with increases in size and endurance. But at a certain point in your fitness journey, you'll need to choose *one* of the outcomes above and tailor your training approach toward reaching that goal. You might even have different goals for different muscle groups. For example, your program could train arms for hypertrophy while training legs for strength.

There are specific approaches required to reach each of these goals. Here they are, along with some reasons why you might choose each one.

TRAINING FOR STRENGTH

Many people assume that when you lift weights you are trying to increase strength. That's only partly true. You might be more concerned with how you look, and the strongest guy isn't necessarily the most *muscular*. An Olympic weightlifter attempting a record for the clean and jerk isn't focused on aesthetics. He isn't as concerned with how his body looks or how lean he is because his goal is to be as strong as possible during this specialized movement. He may even neglect muscles that don't help with competition because he trains exclusively for *strength*.

People have asked me how some guys at the gym with less perceived muscle size can lift way heavier weights than other guys who appear to be jacked. That's because **muscle strength isn't wholly reliant on muscle development**. How strong you are is also determined by the strength and stability of your joints, the length of your muscles, and the ratio of *fast-twitch muscle fibers* (muscles that are used in powerful bursts of movement) to *slow-twitch muscle fibers* (muscles that are used in long-endurance activities). All of these things are genetically predetermined.

How to Train for Strength

Typically, training for strength means working in a lower rep range—generally one to six reps—at 90% of your one-rep max. A common approach to a strength-building set is the "5x5":

5 reps x 5 sets of an exercise at 90% of your one-rep max.

The Benefits of Training for Strength

Training for strength is great, but it might not be your goal. You may be more concerned with building a balanced, athletic, lean physique. If so, you might not care how much weight you can move. *And that's okay!* But don't discount the benefits of training for strength.

Increased strength benefits you in several ways. First of all, training for strength is a *neuromuscular* approach. When you lift the heaviest weights possible, you train your nervous system to recruit more of your existing muscle fibers during each contraction to complete the movement. This is called *neural drive*. Instead of engaging the muscle fibers you typically engage during everyday activities, training for strength forces your body to engage more of your existing muscle fibers to move the weight, including fibers that aren't routinely active. You train your body to use all the muscle tissue it has, instead of the bare minimum amount it needs day-to-day. Training for strength therefore increases neural drive.[69]

Training for strength also increases your musculoskeletal coordination. By moving the heaviest weight possible, your bones, connective tissues, and joints also engage in ways they don't usually work on the daily. Training for strength teaches those parts of your body to practice their usefulness, which makes easy movements even easier movements.

Training for strength goes hand in hand with training for hypertrophy. If your main goal is to get bigger, these two things—better neural drive and better coordination—will improve your hypertrophy workouts, because greater muscle efficiency and engagement means more productive workouts overall.

> **Training for strength is an integral part of any training regimen, no matter your goals.**

Training for Strength During a Fat-Loss Phase

Training for strength while attempting a caloric deficit helps you to maintain the muscle mass you have without overly increasing metabolic activity. In simple terms, training for strength doesn't burn as many calories as other approaches. While training for strength is generally a neuromuscular approach, training for hypertrophy or endurance encourages more metabolic activity. Hypertrophy and endurance workouts fire up your metabolism, which causes you to burn more calories. That makes you hungry, thus making it harder to maintain the deficit you've already created. For this reason, training for strength is often the approach taken by people on a restricted-calorie diet.

That said, I don't recommend training exclusively for strength if you are new to all of this. In general, you can't increase muscle mass while in a caloric deficit because you need excess calories to build muscle. But for newbies, the calories you consume are *redirected* toward muscle growth for the first time, making it easier to gain muscle while also losing fat. Those people may experience gains in size while losing fat, so a combination of approaches is best.

But for those with experience, training for strength helps you hold on to muscle while cycling through a fat-loss phase. And because the exercise is less metabolic, it's less likely to turn you into a Hungry, Hungry Hippo.

TRAINING FOR HYPERTROPHY (SIZE)

Hypertrophy is an increase in the volume of an organ—here, specifically, an increase in the *size* of your muscles. Multiple factors determine muscle size:

- The number of fibers in the muscle;
- The size of each fiber;
- The amount of glycogen and water stored in the muscle; and
- The size of the surrounding muscles and connective tissues.

Leanness—a lack of fat surrounding the muscle—can also increase its *perceived* size. That's because greater muscle definition increases our perception of the individual muscle. All other factors equal, two pounds of lean muscle appear bigger than two pounds of muscle surrounded by fat, even though it's the same amount of muscle. This is why I recommend that you lose the fat first.*

Increasing Muscle Size

If your goal is to increase muscle size, then you will use a hypertrophic approach. You will attempt to tear down the muscle fibers—in other words, break them—which leads to growth after muscle repair. When muscle fibers break, inflammation around the busted cells prompts your body to increase the size of the cells that remain, making them more resistant to future stress.

---

* I wrote an article about this topic. Check it out at fitnrd.com/fatfirst.

In general, hypertrophy in adult humans is not an increase in the *number* of fibers in your muscles. In fact, "growth in cell numbers is limited to the prenatal and immediately postnatal period," and people are "born with or soon reaching their full complement of muscle cells."[70]

Hypertrophy is an increase in the size of *individual cells* within your muscle fibers. Increases in sarcoplasmic fluid, as well as an increase in myofibrils, contribute to the increase in cell size. Myofibrils are elongated contractile threads of *proteins*, connected to form filaments that make up muscle fibers. (They are fibers *inside* muscle fibers. It's *Fiber-ception*.**) The calories you consume—specifically proteins—are used to build myofibrils.

This increase in muscle size happens over days, weeks, and eventually years following repeated workouts. The process takes time, which is why most people only experience noticeably quick gains when they first begin training. For the rest of us it takes years to add significant muscle mass.

While training for strength aims for immediate results—you lift the heaviest weight you possibly can—training for hypertrophy produces results *later*, after muscle repair occurs.

How to Train for Hypertrophy

Studies show that a higher rep range encourages muscles to add sarcomeres (the structural elements in myofibril) as well as sarcoplasmic fluid. Increasingly higher muscle growth occurs along with increasingly higher training volumes[71] *up to a point*. This increase occurs after a muscle exhausts the ATP energy system and begins to rely on glycogen for fuel. In other words, the process moves from being *anaerobic* toward being *partially aerobic*, sort of like cardiovascular exercise.

> Training for hypertrophy requires a higher rep
> range than training for strength, typically
> eight to 12 reps for three to five sets.

In these higher rep ranges, the body increases blood flow to the muscle to shuttle oxygen there, which facilitates the energy expenditure it needs for these reps post-ATP. The extra blood pushed to your muscles after a hypertrophic set creates the "pump" you might notice during a workout.

** Like the movie *Inception*. Get it?

However, performing more than 12 reps per set moves the exercise further into the aerobic zone with a diminishing rate of return on potential muscle growth.

TRAINING FOR ENDURANCE

The more aerobic an exercise becomes, the more it trains those muscles for *endurance*. Once your sets move past the 12-rep range, you are training for endurance.

Similar to cardiovascular endurance, muscular endurance equates to the amount of time your muscles can endure stress. When training a muscle for endurance, you force it to perform under tension for an extended time, teaching the muscle to resist fatigue for longer periods. You increase the muscle's potential for time under tension because you've accustomed it to a longer duration needed to complete more repetitions.

How to Train for Endurance?

People often choose a rep range between 13 and 25 repetitions when training for endurance. You increase the time under tension by increasing the number of reps. *More reps means more time.* Alternatively, you could also use a slower tempo to increase your time under tension, as this also increases endurance.

Use lighter weights when training for endurance. We know that the total volume you lift is a multiplication of weight per rep times the number of reps. In my experience, the total volume you can move successfully for any exercise is relatively *fixed*. For example, if you can lift 20 pounds five times (a total volume of 100 pounds), you can most likely lift five pounds 20 times. Since 20 repetitions would take longer to complete than five repetitions (with tempo being equal), training with the former approach should improve your endurance.

As so, if you plan to train for greater muscular endurance, first consider the total volume you can lift in a strength-building set at 90% of your max effort. Decide how many reps you want to "endure" for in this endurance set. Then calculate the weight you will use for those reps by dividing the total volume you can lift in the comparable strength set by the higher rep range. Challenge yourself by increasing the number of reps, or increasing the weight in very small amounts.

When to Train for Endurance

Professional athletes weight train for endurance to prepare themselves for their specific sport. For instance, a long-distance runner might use endurance-focused weight training for his legs to increase their longevity under duress. Instead of merely preparing by running as long and as fast as possible, the distance runner also incorporates a workout routine that increases muscle endurance in the primary muscles they use to compete. This would include weightlifting sets in higher rep ranges. (Conversely, a competitive sprinter might train for strength since they aim to move as fast as possible under short-term conditions.)

SUPERSETS

A superset is when you combine two different exercises by doing them back-to-back with no rest between them. This is an advanced technique and unnecessary for most people when they are just starting out. Still, some plans call for them (including some of the plans I've developed) and it's important to understand how doubling up on reps impacts your goals.

A superset will often include two exercises that target the same muscle. They may combine a compound lift with an isolation exercise (e.g., a set of squats followed immediately by leg extensions). Remember that the total number of reps you perform without rest will impact the way your body fuels that work. More reps moves the work into an aerobic zone, even if the exercises are different.

If your goal is to gain size or strength, be careful with supersets. If you decide to incorporate them into your routine, lifting in a lower rep range (less than eight reps) for both exercises is best. Otherwise the combined total repetitions move you into the endurance range, which may stifle your potential for growth.

FINAL THOUGHT

The total volume of weight you can lift in an exercise is approximately fixed. These three training methods differ solely by the amount of time you spend lifting that fixed amount of weight, and that time is most easily increased by increasing the number of repetitions. The more repetitions you use to move that fixed volume, the more aerobic the exercise becomes. The more aerobic an exercise, the more it conditions the muscle to endure stress for longer periods.

Because I'm focused on making size and strength gains, **I rarely exceed 12 reps in a set;** the most I will do is 15, including supersets. I expect most people reading this book are looking for similar results. If you want to create a lean, *muscular* physique, avoid excessive endurance training.

I typically begin a workout with one or two compound lifts in a low rep range (less than six). After my muscles begin to fatigue, I move on to several sets in the hypertrophic range (8–12). These sets typically include one or two more compound exercises, followed by one or two isolation exercises. If I plan to train a secondary muscle as an add-on, I will add one or two more isolation exercises to complete the workout.

Below is an example of a typical back and biceps routine.

Example: Back & Biceps Workout:

Pull-up (weighted or assisted, as needed)*	5 sets	4–6 reps
Deadlift*	5 sets	4–6 reps
Lat Pull-down*	5 sets	4–6 reps
Lat Pull-over**	4 sets	8–12 reps
Reverse Fly**	4 sets	8–12 reps
Preacher Curl**	4 sets	8–12 reps
Reverse Dumbbell Curls**	4 sets	8–12 reps

*Strength set   **Hypertrophic set*

THE TAKEAWAY

CHAPTER 21: *STRENGTH, HYPERTROPHY, OR ENDURANCE?*

There are three main approaches to weight training:

» Training for **strength**: You accomplish this with heavier weights and fewer repetitions, typically in the 1–6 rep range at 90% of your maximum effort.

» Training for **hypertrophy** (an increase in size): You accomplish this with moderately heavy weights over 8–12 repetitions.

» Training for **endurance** (increasing the amount of time a muscle can endure stress): You accomplish this with lighter weights in a higher rep range, between 13 and 20 (or more) repetitions.

If your primary goal is fat loss, then I suggest combining both strength sets and hypertrophy sets in your workouts:

» Training for strength helps you to maintain the muscle you have without burning too many calories, which assists you while attempting a caloric deficit. Prioritize this approach if you are experienced and can't expect any muscle growth during a fat-loss phase.

» Training for hypertrophy *may* lead to size increases during a fat-loss phase for those who are new to weight training.

I typically begin a training session by training for strength, and I generally begin with compound exercises. These sets increase neural drive and overall coordination. If you train for strength at the top of a workout, you exhaust the supply of ATP in your muscles. Subsequent hypertrophic sets are even more productive because the process is semi-aerobic from the beginning of the set.

Dedicating a portion of your workouts to hypertrophy or endurance training mimics steady-state, "fat-burning" cardiovascular exercise, like jogging on the treadmill.

If your main goal is to maintain a caloric deficit, you should train mostly in a lower rep range, because higher rep ranges will likely make you hungry:

(continued from previous page)

» I add hypertrophy sets *after* strength sets, toward the back half of my workout, to completely wear out my muscles. My hypertrophic sets are a mix between compound exercises and isolation exercises.

» Your very first reps in these sets should be challenging because the muscle is already fatigued. (I often lose my breath during a hypertrophy workout. My heart rate increases even though I am moving lighter weights.)

CHAPTER 22

CHECK YOUR FORM!

If you make a mistake and do not correct it, this is called a mistake.

CONFUCIUS

Have you ever seen someone in your gym using a machine for the wrong exercise? Have you ever watched a meathead throw a barbell around in a herky-jerky motion, grunting and screaming to draw attention to himself? There are always a few of these people in every gym. They have no idea what they're doing but they also want everyone else to know about it.

How do those folks differ from the guys and gals who seem to know what they're doing? What do you notice when looking at the people with the best physiques? Do they dangerously throw weights around? Do they misuse machines?

Of course not.

Pay attention the next time you're in the gym. The people who've achieved the muscle growth you want, in classic proportions, are focused and intent. They perform each rep correctly, above all else.

They train *methodically*, with highly controlled motions. They use machines for their intended purpose.

They have great form.

FORM FIRST!

Using proper form to challenge your muscles is the entire purpose of strength training. Good form is vital to successful muscle growth. You're in the gym to train specific muscles and muscle groups. Proper form ensures you actually do that, instead of *something else*.

Your form in the gym distinguishes weight training from the everyday movements you make in the real world.

For example, if you need to retrieve a massive box of Christmas decorations from a shelf, you might reach up to grab it and pull it down with your shoulders, then use your back muscles to lower it to chest height, then flex your biceps to carry it across the room, before finally squatting (or bending at the waist if you're not paying attention) to set it down on the floor. You don't *think* about each of those movements as they happen. You don't consciously try to make those moves *harder* for your muscles. You just want to move the damn box as quickly and efficiently as possible.

Efficiency is *not* your goal in the gym. You are there to purposefully challenge your muscles with every movement. You are there to move in an *unconventional* way, beyond your comfort zone.

Using proper form is how you achieve that.

Don't merely try to move the damn weight. You are intentionally making it harder for your muscles to perform these movements, so that each muscle you train that day is stressed beyond what it's accustomed to. You want to push them to their highest potential and, this way, encourage them to grow to surpass that level next time.

You can't make quality gains by rushing through a bunch of garbage reps.* You must control your movements with precision during an exercise to establish accuracy in measuring levels. You do that by mastering the form of each exercise.

The moment you disregard form is the moment you stop training your muscles. Without proper form, there is little difference between strength training and your daily activities. Proper form leads to real gains.

Here are several suggestions to keep in mind as you attempt to master the form during each repetition.

---

* Hurried, unfocused reps with poor form are called "garbage reps." Garbage reps do very little for you, and they're a recipe for injury.

SLOW. IT. DOWN.

Your workout isn't a race. Strength training shouldn't be a high-intensity cardio exercise, and you shouldn't race against a clock. *Don't rush.* If you are short on time, cut out entire exercises. Don't sacrifice your form on one exercise to get to the next one quicker. Save that exercise for your next workout.

I see lots of people in the gym lifting too fast. Spastic movements. Shaky balance. It happens often on cable machines. They grab the rope for a triceps pushdown, and then they push it down as fast as they can, without paying attention to contracting their triceps. Their posture goes to shit. They scrunch their shoulders up to their ears because they're using their back. They don't complete a full range of motion. Instead, they push the rope halfway down, flailing their elbows out wildly, and then they let the weight snap their hands up for the return, completely neglecting the eccentric motion.

That is serious malarkey. Triceps pushdowns are not a back or shoulder exercise! When you scrunch your shoulders, bend your back, and shortcut the full range of motion in pursuit of a speedy set, you cheat your triceps by using other muscles and momentum to throw the weight around.

Why bother doing a triceps exercise if you aren't going to train your triceps?

Your goal in a triceps pushdown—an isolation exercise—is to isolate your triceps. You aren't merely trying to move the rope as quickly as possible. You're deliberately trying to stress your triceps, so your triceps should be the only muscle group working in a triceps pushdown.

This focus applies to every type of exercise, including compound movements. Slow it down, and make sure to engage the appropriate muscle or muscles correctly. If you've been lifting for years with little to show for it, you might be training too fast. *Slow it down!*

LOWER THE WEIGHT

If your form falters, *use less weight on your next set.*

For example, if you can't perform that triceps pushdown correctly—with full extension, without using your shoulders or your back, and with a controlled return—then you need to try the exercise with less weight. If you can't maintain strict control of the motion, with exacting attention to the muscles you are training, then you are lifting more weight than you should be. *Cut it out!*

There is no prize for pushing the heaviest weight in the gym. (Unless you are an Olympian, and I respectfully assume that you aren't). If you work correctly, you make gains over time. That's the prize.

If you work incorrectly, with poor form, you might not make any gains at all. You might even get injured. There are no prizes for injury, either.

Your goal when performing any exercise is to fatigue the targeted muscles. Theoretically, you could do that with a very small amount of weight—or even just your body weight. All muscles can reach fatigue under added resistance *of any amount*. There is no benefit to sacrificing the focus of that resistance to increase the number on the bar or machine.

If your form is anything less than perfect, decrease the weight and try again.

USE DROP SETS

Drop sets are sets of exercises in which you drop the weight progressively after a certain number of reps within the same set. (By "drop" I mean reduce. Don't literally drop the weight.) A drop set is similar to a superset, except the exercise remains the same. This method is excellent for achieving fatigue without sacrificing form.

Let's say your goal is to work in the 12-rep range. You might start at 60% of your max effort for the first six reps and then reduce that to 50% for the second six reps. On a triceps pushdown, that might look like six reps at 60 pounds, then another six reps at 50 pounds.

Reducing the weight mid-set allows you to maintain tension without sacrificing form. The amount of resistance changes, but the time factor remains constant.

It's easier to reduce the weight quickly when training with machines or dumbbells. Drop sets aren't always convenient if you're working with barbells because switching plates takes time. I typically work compound barbell movements for strength early in my routines, and then aim for hypertrophy with dumbbells and machines toward the end when it's easier to incorporate drop sets if my muscles are spent.

You don't need to preplan drop sets to incorporate them into your training. As soon as your form suffers, drop the weight before you try another rep. Keep dropping the weight until you've completed the number of reps you're aiming for in this set while also maintaining proper form. This way, you achieve your target number of reps, instead of stopping short or continuing by squeezing out garbage reps. Drop sets are always an option when proper form becomes impossible during a set.

REMEMBER THE NEGATIVE PORTION OF THE REP

The eccentric, or "negative," portion of a rep is when many people let their form go to shit. That's the segment of the rep when you return the weight to your muscle's extended (i.e., resting) shape. It's easy to sacrifice form during the eccentric movement, especially when you use machines with cables or pulleys. Instead of controlling the weight by using the muscle to return to the starting position, you accidentally let gravity pull it back into place for you. Your hands just go along for the ride.

That's a missed opportunity. Try to maintain a contraction in the muscle even as the muscle lengthens back to the starting position. If you don't control the weight for the second half of the rep, you lose half of the potential benefit of that exercise.

There is no benefit to releasing control of the weight unless your goal is to make a loud sound or to break the equipment. *Hint: it isn't.*

MAINTAIN FOCUS DURING THE PAUSE

Pay attention during the pauses in each rep. Pauses typically occur at the top, midpoint, and end of the repetition. Stay engaged during the moment when your muscle switches gears between movements. *Don't lose focus.* Maintain the contraction during the pauses.

On a bench press, for example, be conscious of your muscles *working* at the top (when you hold the bar above you with arms extended) and at the bottom of the rep (when the bar is lowered at your chest). Feel your chest muscles contracted at these moments, even though they aren't moving. Don't just balance the bar or lock your joints to hold it in position, no matter how brief that pause is.

Even though you rest at the top of the rep, don't *really* rest. The intended muscles should retain control of the weight at all points during the rep, even during pauses. Control is vital not only for TUT but also to prevent injury.

ASK FOR HELP

If you're unsure about proper form, ask for help! There's no shame in getting it right. In my experience, people with good form *love* to talk about their form. Ask someone with experience to spot you, and then politely pick their brain about your technique. Just remember this: never let anyone—even a professional trainer—convince you to lift heavier weights than you are comfortable lifting. It's not worth the risk.

If you are an absolute newbie to the gym, *congratulations!* I highly suggest hiring a personal trainer or enlisting a knowledgeable friend to help you find your bearings. Most gyms offer a free training session when you join, and, if not, it's worth paying for a few sessions to learn how to perform the major exercises with proper form.

If you've been around a while, consider hiring someone to check your form anyway. Any decent trainer will be available for a single session to help you improve your technique on specific exercises or to tweak your approach to certain muscle groups. Some trainers may even help you out for free, just to prove to you that they know what they're doing. It never hurts to ask.

Worst case, *GOOGLE that shit!* There are an infinite number of videos and articles online to help you learn how to perform exercises correctly. Sure, some of it is bullshit, but if the video or article focuses on *safety* or the common mistakes people make, it's probably a good bet.

Even if you've been lifting for years, it never hurts to take a deep dive into videos and tips before you recommit yourself to a new training program. There is always something new to learn, and mastering form is a lifelong pursuit. Plus, it's part of the fun of strength training.

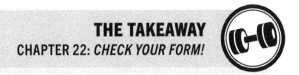

THE TAKEAWAY
CHAPTER 22: *CHECK YOUR FORM!*

Proper form is essential for increasing the size and strength of your muscles. Your form is what distinguishes strength training from your everyday movements outside the gym. Great form ensures your safety and leads to faster gains.

Don't rush. There is no benefit to speeding through reps. You sacrifice time under tension and risk injury when you rush. If you are in a hurry to finish your workout, skip entire exercises.

If your form is less than perfect, lower the weight! You can exhaust any muscle with even a tiny amount of resistance, so long as you maintain a contraction in the muscle. Lifting too heavy encourages mistakes, like utilizing extraneous muscles or momentum to perform the motion.

Use "drop" sets. No, dropping the weight doesn't mean literally dropping the weight onto the floor. It means reducing the amount of weight you're working with in the middle of a set. Drop sets are crucial for maintaining form if you find yourself faltering in the middle of a set.

Don't forget the negative (eccentric) portion of an exercise. Don't use gravity to return to the starting position. Proper form means maintaining a contraction in the muscles on the return motion and thereby controlling the weight at all times.

Stay focused during pauses in a rep. Losing focus leads to abandoning the tension in the muscle and relying on balance or other muscles to hold the weight. You aren't performing this exercise to learn how to balance the bar by locking your elbows! Good form entails holding tension in the target muscles throughout the rep, even during the pauses.

If you aren't 100% certain that you are training with proper form, ask for help. Hire a trainer or ask a friendly expert for advice. Google the exercise to read tips and watch videos about proper technique. Look for videos that prioritize safety. Don't just guess about your form: do the research and ask for help. If help isn't available, consider a different exercise.

CHAPTER 23

THE MIND-MUSCLE CONNECTION

The mind is everything; what you think you become.

ANONYMOUS

MIND OVER MATTER

Now I'm going to go a little deeper with regard to your form. What I'm about to say may seem esoteric, but you can handle it. I want to share a mental strategy that's transformed the way I push weights around the gym. It's called "maintaining the mind-muscle connection."

Maintaining the mind-muscle connection means keeping complete mental focus on the muscle or muscles that you are training during an exercise.

It sounds super simple, but most of us struggle to do it, myself included. I'm easily distracted in the gym.

What's that song they're playing?

What the hell is that guy wearing? And why?

What's happening on Instagram?

Whoa! Look how big my arms look!

Also, they need to fix the pad on this machine...

Despite the simplicity of my routines, I still fight to pay attention to each movement during an exercise. My mind likes to wander...

But I know that I see better results when I really concentrate on the specific muscles I am training during any given exercise. My aim is to focus on that muscle and ignore everything else. It's almost like turning each rep into a meditation or a mindfulness practice. I try to remove all extraneous thoughts from my brain except for one: **to feel the muscle contract.**

You have one task during each rep, and that is to concentrate on the exact muscle you are working, to feel it contract during each rep.

Every Movement Begins in Your Brain

Here's the order of operations when you lift a dumbbell (or any other weight):

- You decide, consciously, to raise the dumbbell;
- Your brain then creates a signal in your nervous system, which prompts the release of acetylcholine* from the nerve endings near the muscles needed to make that motion happen; and then
- The muscle contracts, creating the movement.

Your body doesn't *know* that you have added resistance against your biceps to force it to grow. Your body only knows that you've told it to move the dumbbell. On the contrary, your body will seek the easiest path to moving that dumbbell quickly because it wants to do things the most natural way possible. If that wasn't the case, your body might run an automatic cycle of muscular contractions while you sleep, just for the sake of automating muscle growth.** But it doesn't, unfortunately. At least not in adults.

During many exercises—especially compound ones—there are both primary and secondary muscle groups at work. Your body wants to distribute the weight whatever way it can to make the movement easier. That might also include enlisting the help of other muscles that you aren't training right now. But maintaining a mind-muscle connection ensures that your body doesn't circumnavigate resistance in the *specific* muscle or muscles you're training at this moment.

---

* Acetylcholine: a neurotransmitter (a compound) that converts the electrical signals in your brain into the chemical process needed to tell the cells in your muscle to contract.

** *Wouldn't that be awesome?*

Here's an example. When you curl your biceps with too much weight you might *subconsciously* do the following to compensate:

- Engage your back muscles to move the dumbbell higher in space;

- Engage your leg muscles to create momentum and "swing" the dumbbell upward;

- Engage your forearm muscles to "curl" the weight at the wrist.

But none of these extraneous movements help to grow your biceps! They are crutches. When you use your back, legs, or forearms to curl the dumbbell, you don't know what percentage of the weight you actually carried with your biceps.

However, if you maintain a mind-muscle connection to your biceps throughout the exercise, you're guaranteed to train your biceps.

The mind-muscle connection helps you to prevent secondary or tertiary muscles and joints from decreasing the resistance you are actively trying to create in a specific muscle. This concept seems simple, but I find that it gets harder and harder to practice as I increase the weight. More weight means more resistance, which also means your body naturally looks for more ways to cheat.

Prioritize Muscles During Compound Exercises

A mind-muscle connection also helps you designate the primary muscles you hope to train during a compound exercise. Compound exercises purposefully rely on secondary muscle groups. For instance, the primary muscles you use when you bench press are your chest muscles, but you must also engage your shoulders and triceps secondarily. Your triceps help power the motion, and your shoulders engage to stabilize the bar.

It's nice to work my triceps and shoulders when I perform a set of bench presses, but that's not the reason I bench. *I bench press to grow my chest.* Maintaining a mind-muscle connection makes that happen.

When I bench, I turn my mind toward my chest muscles. I think about my chest, and then I *feel* my chest muscles contract—squeezing together—to move the weight. I visualize my chest muscles working with each rep, and I imagine that I am able to put all of the resistance against my chest muscles. I see myself holding the weight in my chest.

It's easy to pile weight onto the bar when all you want to do is move it. But if your goal is to build your chest muscles, then you want to maintain a mind-muscle connection to your chest to activate and engage those muscles.

Plus, if you focus on stressing the correct muscles, you won't need as much weight to wear them out. Some athletes swear that they can fatigue their muscles with very little or no weight at all, just by engaging the muscle and creating resistance with their mind.

But what if you are benching to train your triceps? That's fine! If so, adjust your grip accordingly (more narrowly in this instance), and root your mind in your triceps. If you concentrate on keeping your triceps muscles flexed and engaged throughout the movement, that's where you'll experience growth.

"But Nate," you might say, "what if I want to use a compound exercise to stimulate growth in *all* of those muscles at the same time?"

Well, you naturally add some resistance to secondary muscles in a compound exercise without maintaining focus on them. But if you truly hope to prioritize those secondary muscles equally while performing the exercise, then you'll need to maintain a mind-muscle connection with *all* of the muscles involved in the exercise simultaneously, or in the sequence they engage. That's possible, but it's not easy for me. I prefer to connect consciously to a single muscle while holding the other muscle groups in the back of my mind. That's how I use the mind-muscle connection to gain size and strength where I want to.

THE TAKEAWAY
CHAPTER 23: *THE MIND-MUSCLE CONNECTION*

Create a mind-muscle connection by consciously focusing on the muscle you're training during each movement in a repetition. Feel the muscle contract, and visualize placing all of the resistance there.

Maintaining a mind-muscle connection during an exercise keeps you focused on proper form and may also increase muscle growth.

Mind over matter. If you think it, growth will come.

CHAPTER 24

TEMPO & REST

As you get the rhythm you discern how to win.

MIYAMOTO MUSASHI, *The Book of Five Rings*

TRAINING WITH TEMPOS

Strength-training tempo indications appear as a series of four numbers next to an exercise (e.g., X-X-X-X). The four digits indicate the time in seconds you spend during each portion of the repetition:

- The first number is the time spent on the eccentric, lengthening motion of the exercise, also called "the negative";

- The second number indicates a pause, if any, at the midpoint;

- The third number is the time spent on the concentric, shortening motion; and

- The fourth number denotes a pause, if any, at the bottom, before you begin the next rep.

Serious lifters often train with complex tempo patterns, but these patterns are unnecessary for most of us. Training plans I see for sale on the Internet often incorporate convoluted tempos as a way to differentiate them from the other training plans out there. Instead of merely telling you which exercises to perform, they also instruct you to "count to five" here or pause for "three seconds" there to distinguish their routine from the norm.

For a newcomer, most of these tempo patterns are too complicated and distracting. The benefits of adjusting the tempo of your reps are to help maintain the mind-muscle connection and to increase time under tension, both of which you can achieve *without* confusing tempo patterns.

Training with complicated tempo patterns is an advanced training method. If you are reading this book, you're most likely a beginner or someone who is concentrated, first and foremost, on burning excess fat. Instead of trying to follow many different tempo patterns for the various exercises in your workout, I suggest using a single tempo pattern that's simple and easy to remember: **2-1-2-1.**

Using the bench press as an example, here's how our 2-1-2-1 tempo looks during each repetition:

a. Hold the bar above you (starting position).
b. Lower the bar to your chest slowly for **a count of two seconds.** During this motion, your pec muscles lengthen.
c. Pause with the bar in the lowered position for **a count of one second.**
d. Raise the bar back to the starting position for **a count of two seconds** while contracting your pec muscles.
e. Finally, **count one second** before lowering the bar again.

Counting to two during both the eccentric and concentric motions forces you to move the weight slowly, with purpose and concentration. You won't drop the bar if you are trying to delay the movement over a count of two. You maintain a mind-muscle connection because you fill that time by focusing on your muscles, and you increase your total time under tension.

If you are a beginner to serious gains, the 2-1-2-1 tempo is a terrific place to start. This tempo slows down your reps and helps you concentrate on the work. It's also easy to remember! When a training program gives you a different tempo for each exercise, it gets super confusing very fast. You count different numbers throughout the rep while also counting reps, and then you have to figure out a different set of numbers for the next exercise, too. Who has time to remember all those numbers? With a 2-1-2-1 pattern, you know that you spend two beats on *both* concentric and eccentric motions, which removes the hassle of remembering how to count while thinking about your muscles.

I recommend you avoid advanced tempo training at first. Stick to a 2-1-2-1 tempo. It's easy to count and delivers equal emphasis to all movements in the rep without having to remember a bunch of numbers.

TIME UNDER TENSION, REVISITED

Let's calculate the TUT of a 2-1-2-1 tempo on the bench. Assuming that I maintain full muscle engagement during both movements and the hold (while the bar is lowered to my chest), I can calculate my total time under tension as follows:

2 sec eccentric contraction

+ 1 sec contracted pause

+ 2 sec concentric contraction

= **5 sec of forced tension on the muscle during each rep**

5 sec tension per rep x 12 reps in the set

= **60 sec of total time under tension for the entire set**

However, if I didn't keep any tempo and I lowered the bar quickly, let it bounce, and then pushed it up fast again, my TUT might look more like this:

0.5 sec eccentric contraction

+ 0 sec contraction in pause (because the bar bounced)

+ 0.5 sec concentric contraction

= **1 sec of forced tension on the muscle during each rep**

1 sec tension per rep x 12 reps

= **12 sec of total time under tension for the set**

That's a huge difference in the amount of time under tension! You can see that a 2-1-2-1 tempo trains your muscles *five times harder* than the half-second tempo.

The second example also assumes full muscle engagement during all motions, even though the bar moved very quickly (0.5 seconds). That's highly unlikely! How could anyone actually concentrate on muscle contraction in half a second? Using a 2-1-2-1 tempo creates ample time under tension and provides you with enough time to focus on form.

REST BETWEEN SETS

Your training tempo also includes the amount of time you rest between sets. I take a simple approach to resting: I *increase* rest time as my rep count *decreases*. Longer sets with lower weights require less rest between sets than shorter sets with heavier weights. Aim for the following rest periods between sets, depending on whether you are performing the exercise for strength, hypertrophy, or endurance.

Resting for Strength

If you are training for strength and attempting to lift heavy, consider a rest time of **two to three minutes between sets.** That might seem like an eternity, but it's necessary to reset and prep for the next explosive set. Strength training in the low rep range (<6 reps + weight at >80% of your one-rep max) relies mainly on the ATP-PC system for energy to complete the motions. This action is purely anaerobic, meaning that it doesn't require oxygen to create energy. It relies on phosphagen stores, which are replenished slowly. Complete phosphagen repletion takes approximately three minutes.[72] When training in a lower rep range for strength increases, it doesn't make sense to cut rest time because the muscle won't be ready to do its job during the next set. Resting for less than two minutes defeats the purpose of this training approach.

Resting for Hypertrophy

If you're training for hypertrophy in an eight- to 12-rep range, then I suggest a rest time of **approximately one minute.** This might be 45 seconds for sets with higher reps (e.g., 12 reps) or one minute 30 seconds for sets on the lower end of that range (e.g., eight reps).

Training for hypertrophy requires a mix of ATP *and* glycogen stores to perform the exercise. Your body is efficient at replenishing glycogen in your muscles through a partially aerobic process. That blood rush to your muscles is more than a pump; it's your body replenishing the glycogen in your muscles. This process doesn't take as long as replenishing ATP, so a shorter rest period accommodates your needs.

Resting for Endurance

Endurance training requires *even shorter* rest periods because it's primarily aerobic. The goal of endurance training is to remain in an aerobic zone for as much time as possible. Resting brings your heart rate down and pulls you out of the zone. If you train for endurance, I suggest a rest time of 30 seconds between sets.

This applies to endurance lifting the same way it might apply to cardio exercises. Because the weight is lower than it would be for strength and hypertrophy training, you can perform more reps before the muscle fatigues. The stress on your muscles builds over *time*, and you don't typically feel it until the end of the set.

The quality of endurance exercise depends on your heart rate, which elevates over the course of the set. When you stop moving, your heart rate slows, and your breathing rate decreases because you aren't shuttling that extra blood to your muscles. Once your breathing returns to a regular cadence, your glycogen reserves are, in theory, restored. Get back to work as soon as you catch your breath.

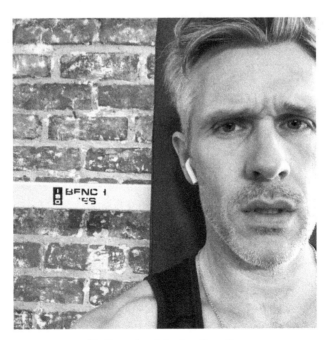

No, I'm not just sitting here. I'm resting.

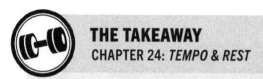

THE TAKEAWAY
CHAPTER 24: *TEMPO & REST*

Counting a tempo during each repetition helps you preserve the mind-muscle connection and forces you to concentrate on maintaining muscle engagement.

Exercise tempo is typically indicated by a string of **four numbers: X-X-X-X.** These numbers represent the time in seconds you spend on each part of the rep:

1. The eccentric contraction

2. The pause between contractions

3. The concentric contraction

4. A pause to reset at the bottom of the repetition

I recommend a 2-1-2-1 tempo for most exercises. It's easy to remember, easy to count, and it slows down the contractions in the rep. All of this increases your time under tension during the set. Avoid experimenting with complicated tempos until you are an expert. *You don't need 'em.*

Increase rest time between sets as rep count increases.

» Fewer reps with heavier weights require longer rest times because it takes longer to restore the ATP (fuel) needed to perform well.

» More reps with lighter weights require shorter rest times because the aerobic process restores the glycogen needed relatively quickly.

Recommended rest periods between sets are as follows:

» When training for **strength** (<6 reps): **2–3 minutes**

» When training for **hypertrophy** (8–12 reps): **1 minute** on average, ranging from 45 seconds to 1 minute, 30 seconds

» When training for **endurance** (13+ reps), minimize rest time between sets: no more than **30 seconds, or until you catch your breath.**

CHAPTER 25

STRETCHING & MOBILITY WORK

A blazing fire makes flame and brightness out of everything that is thrown into it.

MARCUS AURELIUS

MY EXPERIENCE WITH BACK PAIN

I broke my back during a diving accident when I was a freshman in college. (Honestly, I was bridge jumping. Do you know that old saying about your friends jumping off a bridge? I learned the hard way.) I had a few compression fractures, and I wore a full-thoracic back brace for several months. But I was very fortunate; if my center of gravity had shifted a bit more and caused me to land higher up my back or on my neck, I might have sustained a much worse injury.

Throughout the rest of my college career, I dedicated myself to making sure that this injury wouldn't catch up with me later in life. I knew that compression fractures could degenerate into debilitating back conditions, so I steadily worked to strengthen my lower back muscles and to stretch my spine every day. It also helped that I was a theater major and had to enroll in lots of dance classes. I'm not much of a dancer, but I used these classes to increase my flexibility and range of motion. I also took yoga, and I still practice yoga regularly as an adult.

A few years ago, I experienced the first real back pain I've ever felt since that injury. I'd had minor pain before, but this was different. Honestly I don't remember how it happened, but one morning I woke up with severe pain and I didn't get out of bed for two days. *It sucked.*

On the third day, I called a chiropractor. Before he would examine me, he sent me for an X-ray so he could assess the current state of the injury I'd sustained in college. Later that week, the results came back, and I hobbled into his office. During that examination he told me several things that changed my life.

First, he explained to me that my activities in college—dance and yoga— had "saved my life." He'd never before seen a compression fracture heal as well as mine had. My spine maintained a normal curve, and he told me that this miraculous healing was due to the stretching and mobility work I did in the years following my injury.

The second thing he said was a major wake-up call. He explained that the back pain I was currently experiencing was unrelated to my previous injury. It had nothing to do with breaking my back all those years ago. The cause, he said, was tightness in my posterior chain, specifically in my hamstrings. My hips were "locked" because I sit so much during the day. Sitting at my desk for hours every day had disproportionately tightened my hamstrings while simultaneously stretching my quads. *I had sprained my back during the simple act of bending over to pick something up.* My hips weren't flexing like they're supposed to, so a muscle in my lower back stretched too far to compensate for the lack of mobility in my hips, and—*pop!*—intense pain for days.

What's worse, I'd likely been straining my back over and over again every time I bent at the waist, because my hips were so tight. It was a vicious cycle. The doctor warned me that it would keep happening unless I stretched my hip flexors and hamstrings. He showed me a few simple stretches, gave me an adjustment to open my hip sockets, and sent me on my way.

Oh my God, he was right.

I started doing those stretches regularly to loosen my hamstrings and open my hips. I limited activities that were tightening my hamstrings—like running or sitting for too long without breaks—and I made sure to strengthen opposing muscle groups. I also started practicing yoga again.

And you know what? *I haven't had any lower back pain in five years.*

BACK PAIN IS A COMMON PROBLEM

My story isn't unique. Approximately 80% of Americans experience lower back pain at some point in their life.[73] Potential causes run the gamut from injury to neglect, from smoking to genetic predisposition.

But one thing is certain: regular stretching prevents or eases chronic back pain. A healthy spine is vital to everything you do, including strength training. Regular stretching is the number one solution for preventing pulls, sprains, twists, and any of the injuries that knock you out of commission.

Increased Mobility Means Less Risk of Injury

Stretching increases mobility, which goes a long way toward preventing chronic back pain and other injuries. If your muscles or connective tissues are too tight in one area, your body tries to compensate for the limited range of motion by engaging superfluous tissue. It attempts to use surrounding muscles to facilitate the movements of muscles and joints that aren't prepared for the task at hand. *But your body isn't engineered to use those other muscles,* so this leads to sprains and strains and tears, or worse.

Stretching equips your body for a full range of motion so that it can work as designed. It also *increases* your comfortable range of motion over time, which further improves mobility. More mobility means less risk of injury.

Stretching Facilitates Muscle Growth

Stretching increases the regular flow of blood to muscles, ligaments, and tendons post-stretch. Your body responds to stretching by ensuring efficient blood flow to those areas even when they are at rest. That blood brings oxygen and nutrients, which leads to healthier muscles and connective tissues that are better prepared to face the rigors of a weightlifting program. Well-oxygenated muscles are better primed for strength training and, ultimately, muscle growth.

Stretching Is an Antidote to Sitting

Sitting at a desk all day is one of the worst things you can do to your body. When we sit, we shorten our hamstrings, we extend our quads, and we lock our hips in an unnatural position. Doing this for hours every day creates a muscular imbalance, and sets us up for injury.

In a study of 447 office workers who sat at their desks for an average of 6.29 hours during an eight-hour workday, the results showed prolonged sitting caused "musculoskeletal disorder symptoms" in the lower back, thighs, knees, and shoulders, among other symptoms like exhaustion and hypertension.[74] Many of us amplify the problem by slumping on a couch in front of the television in the evening. If you experience chronic back, neck, or shoulder pain, there is a high probability that it is caused by sitting for prolonged periods.

Stretching counteracts the damage caused by routine sitting. A consistent stretching regimen corrects musculoskeletal imbalances, lessening the pain and maybe even removing it altogether. If you suffer from minor aches and pains—or worse—you probably need to start stretching!

INCORPORATE REGULAR STRETCHING

Dedicate at least 30 minutes, two or three times a week, to stretching and mobility work. *Schedule time to stretch*, and be consistent. Your stretching sessions should be independent of your other workouts. Take a yoga class or follow along with stretching videos on Facebook. (Yes, this is a thing.) Make sure to stretch the areas where you hold tension. If you primarily work at a seated desk, find time to stand up and stretch gently throughout the workday.

I also suggest you find a professional who can assess your current mobility, posture, and address any regular pain you experience. They can show you stretches that apply to your specific concerns, and teach you how to do them at home in your spare time.

So, *how* do you find a professional?

Take a yoga class. Take a Pilates class. Schedule a session with a trainer who incorporates stretching into their routine. There are studios that specialize in mobility training popping up everywhere,[75] and many strip-mall chain massage parlors offer stretching options now. *Get on it!*

Once you know what to do, make time to do it. Stretch on the floor while you're watching television in the evening.

Invest in Your Future

In terms of aging without pain, stretching is even more important than strength training. You cannot build the body you want while enduring regular pain. Posture, balance, and basic mobility are the foundation of your entire physical being. If you skip stretching, then you're gambling with your future health. No, you don't need to become a yoga guru. But you do need to make sure your muscles are limber and poised to support you for the rest of your life. You can learn to stretch at any age, and it will always help to prepare you for the years ahead.

Should You Stretch After a Workout?

Yes, I stretch briefly after almost every strength-training workout. I use foam rollers to massage my iliotibial (IT) bands, and I use a wall to stretch my hamstrings. I practice extending my posterior chain—namely my hamstrings and glutes—after almost every workout, no matter what body parts I trained that day. I'm not talking about a full-on mat session; I just put my hands on a wall and stretch my hamstrings. These stretches take me less than two minutes. I save my progressive stretch training work for class situations when I'm focused on *increasing* mobility.

I also stretch both before and after cardiovascular exercise, especially if I'm running or jogging. Many high-impact activities, like running, rely on fast-twitch muscle responses. If you jerk these muscles around while they are cold, you increase the risk of a strain or sprain during the activity. I stretch briefly beforehand to increase blood flow to those muscles, and again afterward to prevent injury. A few minutes is usually enough.

Figure out what works for you, preferably with the guidance of a professional, then make stretching a regular habit. Everyone benefits from stretching and mobility work of some kind. *Don't skip it!*

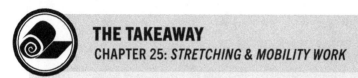

THE TAKEAWAY
CHAPTER 25: *STRETCHING & MOBILITY WORK*

Stretching is vital to both your fitness journey and your long-term health.

» Regular stretching addresses many forms of back pain and prevents further injury. Additionally, stretching increases blood flow to the muscles and connective tissues you use during strength training.

» Sitting all day wreaks havoc on your muscles and connective tissues. Adding weightlifting to the mix creates a recipe for muscular imbalance. That leads to aches and pains you won't see coming until it's too late.

Improved mobility counterbalances the many ways we passively abuse our bodies every day.

» Regularly stretching your posterior chain can significantly decrease your risk of future back pain. If you are among the 80% of Americans who have or will experience lower back pain, then stretching is your antidote.

Stretch in conjunction with other exercise:

» Add a few minutes of light stretching after every strength-training session.

» Stretch before and after a cardio workout, like running or biking. Warming up your muscles prior to high-impact exercises will help prevent sprains and strains during the activity.

Dedicate time to progressive stretching sessions outside of your weightlifting routine.

» Incorporate a program to *increase* your mobility, like a yoga or Pilates class, or by working with a stretching coach or trainer.

CHAPTER 26

HOW MANY DAYS PER WEEK?
(STRENGTH-TRAINING SPLITS)

*There is virtue in work and there is virtue in rest.
Use both and overlook neither.*

ALAN COHEN

BUILDING REST DAYS INTO YOUR ROUTINE

The number of days you train each week is known as your *strength-training split*. Your split depends mainly on how many times per week you plan to target each muscle group, and how much time you'll need to rest your muscles in between training sessions.

I believe in scheduling a split around rest days to avoid the possibility of overtraining. Rest is *vital* for muscle growth, especially during a hypertrophic approach. You *need* rest days to reach your goals. You *must* schedule rest days as part of your routine.

Think of rest days as *growth days* because that's when your muscles actually grow. When you strength train, you try to wear out your muscles—to break them down—so that they come back bigger and stronger. But if you continuously tear down your muscles by overtraining, they never have a chance to regenerate.

It's easy to forget this when starting a new fitness program. You're excited about diving in and getting results. That energy and commitment are necessary for success, but it's common to try to *overtrain* when you are obsessed.

When you continuously concentrate on your fitness goals, rest days make you restless. Time away from the gym might feel counterproductive, but you've got to fight that feeling. Overtraining is unlikely to increase your gains, and more often leads to injury and fatigue.

Unless you have a unique genetic predisposition for muscle growth and very flexible schedule, **training more than four or five times per week doesn't give your muscles enough time to recoup.** Some professionals recommend training no more than four times per week, or for more than two days in a row.[76] There are 6-day splits and methods for hitting every major muscle group three times per week, but how could you expect to manage that while also maintaining a caloric deficit? (Not to mention *living your life.*) If fat loss is your first priority, you need rest just as much as you need to train.

Additionally, several studies indicate that reducing training frequency has little effect on results, up to a point. Obviously not training *at all* yields no benefit, but the change in benefit from reducing frequency from two or three times per week to once per week may be marginal for most people,[77] with the benefits of once- or twice-per-week sessions still being enough to maintain strength.[78] And research on the effect of training volume on growth also indicates that training for less than an hour produced similar results to training five times that amount.[79]

All of that is to say that how often you train is less important than *how hard* you train. Increased volume during fewer workouts will likely yield similar results to training more frequently with less volume per set. And the more often you train, the more difficult it becomes to train *hard*, especially while maintaining a caloric deficit. Training each body part with 15–25 sets per week provides more than enough stimulus for hypertrophy. More than 25 sets in a week may prove to be futile.

Sure, it may feel productive to hit the gym every day this week or for a second time today, but it's not worth the frustration you'll feel in two months when you haven't made any gains. Unless building muscle is your full-time job (it's not) you should prioritize sleep, stretching, and downtime over all those extra workouts. Spending all that time in the gym is an unsustainable approach for modern folks with jobs and families. Training too much will wear you out, and you'll be more likely to abandon your goals.

Here are a few tips to build a split that prioritizes rest, fits into your lifestyle, and keeps you motivated even on days you aren't lifting weights.

REST MUSCLE GROUPS AS PART OF YOUR SPLIT

Remember to rest muscle groups between workouts, even when you go to the gym on consecutive days. **Give specific muscles 48 hours or more to recuperate before training them again.** For example, you shouldn't work your chest two days in a row. Resting your chest doesn't preclude you from working your legs, back, abs, or biceps, so you still have plenty of muscle groups to work the next day. You might even be able to isolate a secondary muscle group—like your shoulders or triceps in this instance—24 hours after you work your chest, as long as you didn't isolate them as part of the chest day routine.

FIVE DAYS, MAX

I don't recommend more than five days of strength training per week while trying to lose fat. A 5-day split is an aggressive approach to weightlifting that allows for two full rest days. When planned correctly, it also gives you time to rest individual muscle groups for two days while consecutive workouts concentrate on other muscle groups. It also leaves plenty of room for both strength and hypertrophy sets every time you hit the gym.

A 5-day split allows for some specialization, too. You'll have extra opportunities to train weak spots repeatedly, two or possibly even three times in a week. For example, I'm pinpointing my legs right now because I'd like a bigger ass... er, I mean I'd like to add mass. I typically work legs for strength on Mondays, with an emphasis on heavy compound movements, like squats. Then I work legs again on Fridays, featuring isolation exercises—like leg extensions and hamstring curls—in hypertrophy rep ranges.

Working legs on both Mondays and Fridays still provides adequate rest; three days after strength exercises (Tuesdays, Wednesdays, and Thursdays) and two days after hypertrophy exercises (Saturdays and Sundays). Some weeks I further differentiate these days by devoting Monday to hamstrings and Friday to quadriceps. A 5-day split makes this possible while also providing ample opportunity to train other muscle groups twice a week, albeit with less intensity than I train my legs.

My Basic 5-Day Split:

Monday: Legs (strength)

Tuesday: Chest, Triceps, & Shoulders

Wednesday: Back & Biceps

Thursday: REST

Friday: Legs (hypertrophy)

Saturday: Upper Body (hypertrophy exercises for chest, biceps, triceps, and shoulders)

Sunday: REST

This split prevents overtraining but also allows me to train each muscle group twice each week. With this split, I give each muscle group at least two days to rest before hitting them again. I also include two full rest days to give my entire muscle-building system a chance to recoup and to prioritize a higher caloric deficit.

Consider a 3- or 4-Day Split

If your primary goal is fat loss, then your training program should support that; a 3- or 4-day split might work better for your fat-loss goals. Shoot for maintaining muscle mass while in a caloric deficit, not for gaining more muscle.

Four days is plenty of time to hit all of the major muscle groups and still include a few isolation exercises to target trouble areas or "vanity" muscles. It also gives you three full days each week in which to engage in a higher caloric deficit.

However, a 3-day split might be *even better* if you have more fat to lose because that split provides you with four days of a higher caloric deficit. You can still train all major muscle groups during a 3-day split. The *push-pull-leg* split is a common approach:

- One day for pushing exercises, training chest, triceps and shoulders;
- One day for pulling exercises to train back and biceps; and
- One day to train legs.

Don't be tempted to train more than you need to. Three days is a great place to start when you're trying to lose fat. You'll experience much faster fat loss by maximizing your deficit for four days each week than you would by training for five days. Pick your priorities and commit to them!

BUILDING THE SPLIT

You might wonder my position on how to group muscles together when building your split. I wish I had a concrete answer for you, but there are too many conflicting opinions and not enough quality research to confidently say that any one of these approaches works better than another.

Some people suggest training *complementary* muscle groups together (e.g., training triceps after chest). Other people suggest training *opposing* muscles together (e.g., training triceps with biceps). Still other splits simply divide the week into upper body and lower body workouts, or *push* and *pull* exercises. Each approach has its place. The only thing I know with certainty is that overtraining stifles progress, so group exercises in a way that maximizes rest.

Here's the good news: with so many strength-training plans available on the Internet now, there is sure to be one that works for your priorities and schedule. I've included my basic plan in this book, and I'll put additional plans online, too. But the best weight-training split is the one that keeps you going back to the gym. The program you choose needs to keep you motivated, safe, and excited to be in the gym.

Personally, I like to mix it up. At this point there aren't many new exercises for me to incorporate into my routines, so I vary my workouts by trying different combinations of exercises on different days. I don't believe that *when* you train a muscle has nearly as much impact on growth as how well you rest that muscle.*

---

* There is evidence that training legs increases testosterone production, and that adding a smaller muscle group to your leg-day workout increases gains for that additional muscle group. I've written an article about this at fitnrd.com/legs in case you're interested in reading more.

DON'T "REST" YOUR GOALS

Remember that every day counts toward your goals, even if it's a rest day. Don't lose sight of your objectives merely because you're not lifting weights. Continue to track calories. Continue to set small goals for the day, even though they aren't gym goals. View your rest day as an opportunity to check in on your progress, to plan the coming days and weeks, and to read up on exercise form or nutrition.

Resist the temptation to overeat on rest days. A day off from the gym is not a day off from your total weekly deficit. Fat loss is a long-term process, and a healthy caloric deficit is only effective over time. Use your rest day to rest your muscles... but don't rest your discipline by eating an entire pizza. Rest days are an opportunity to increase your caloric deficit to the max (i.e., eating at or just above your BMR). It's much easier to increase your deficit on a day that you aren't lifting weights, because lifting days require a higher level of calories to fuel your workout.

You might also consider adding cardio exercise on rest days. I often use rest days to program long, slow cardio, such as a three-mile walk or a comfortable bike ride. This sort of exercise burns a few extra calories but doesn't tax the muscles I'm resting.

Sometimes I add high-intensity cardio work on a rest day, but I try not to push myself too hard. Don't do high-impact cardio that stresses a muscle group you just trained. For example, don't do sprint intervals the day after you work your legs. I train legs at the beginning of the week to give them a break from strength training before I hit them with cardio on a rest day (typically Thursdays). I can jog or swim or bike on a rest day without feeling my quads turn into Jell-O.

You should also consider programming mobility work on rest days. Take a gentle yoga class, or devote a full 30 minutes to stretching. Scheduling slow, static stretching routines on your rest days provides you with a dedicated window for including stretching as a part of your program. Alternatively, a "flow" yoga class raises your heart rate a bit while also accomplishing your mobility quota for the week. Whatever you do, avoid *active* stretching which may lead to overtraining your muscles while they recoup from strength training. Concentrate on posture, balance, joint health, and essential flexibility. Use these stretching sessions to ensure that your strength-training sessions aren't tightening you up in ways that can lead to injury.

THE TAKEAWAY
CHAPTER 26: *HOW MANY DAYS PER WEEK?*

Prioritize rest days when choosing a weightlifting split. Rest days are essential for muscle growth, so resist the temptation to skip them. Overtraining is unlikely to increase your gains, and more often leads to injury and fatigue.

If you are serious about gaining muscle, I recommend a 5-day training split, which includes two rest days each week. Five training days per week provide plenty of time to work all of your muscle groups twice, with variations in compound movements, isolation exercises, and sets geared toward both strength and hypertrophy.

A 4-day or 3-day split may be more advantageous for fat loss. It's easier to maintain a significant caloric deficit on rest days. Three or even four days of eating close to your BMR while resting can make a massive difference in your total caloric deficit for the week. Plus, training three times per week gives you plenty of time to target every muscle in your body.

Avoid overtraining. If your goal is hypertrophy, aim for 15–25 sets per muscle group each week.

When programming your split, **group muscles according to your priorities.** There isn't enough concrete evidence to support favoring one method of combining muscle groups over another. Combining complementary muscles, opposing muscles, or grouping by *push* and *pull* movements are all good strategies. Do what works for you and your schedule!

A rest day is *not* a break from your fitness goals.

» Don't neglect your caloric deficit on rest days. Use the downtime to check in on progress, review nutrition and exercise concepts, and plan for the days ahead.

» Schedule easy cardio on rest days, like a long walk or a casual bike ride. These activities increase your caloric burn for the day without taxing the muscles you are resting.

» Add a stretching or mobility routine to your dedicated rest days. Take a gentle yoga class or stretch passively in front of the television.

PART FOUR:
CARDIO

CHAPTER 27

THE REAL PURPOSE OF CARDIO

To what goal are you straining? The whole future lies in uncertainty: live immediately.

SENECA

CARDIO: THE BENEFITS

Cardiovascular exercise is physical movement that relies primarily on the cardiovascular system. We're talking about your heart, lungs, and pulmonary network. As a cardio exercise increases in intensity, your body requires *more* oxygen to perform, meaning you breathe harder and your heart pumps faster to deliver that oxygen to your muscles.

The true purpose of cardio exercise is to improve your cardiovascular response—that is, the efficiency and performance of your heart and lungs.

Self-explanatory, yeah? Unfortunately, many people have been tricked into thinking that cardiovascular exercise is the best way to lose fat. Spoiler alert: *cardio is not the best way to lose fat.* More on that in the next chapter, but first let me explain some of the many benefits of improving your cardiovascular system through cardio exercise.

General Health

A healthy heart is like an insurance policy against heart disease or malfunction, but that's not all. When your heart functions efficiently, that efficiency benefits every other part of your body. More oxygen to your brain means better cognitive performance and less likelihood of dementia later in life. More oxygen shuttled to your muscles means faster recovery after strength training, better recovery after illness, and better sleep. It improves your immune system. Plus, cardiovascular exercise may lessen your risk of osteoporosis, diabetes, and some forms of cancer.[80] The list goes on.

VO2 Max

Cardio training increases your VO2 max, which is the maximum amount of oxygen your body can process under duress. Ever notice that you breathe deeper during cardiovascular exercise? Your lungs expand further than normal so that your body can process the oxygen it needs during that run or swim or bike ride. Practicing that expansion increases your VO2 max.

Increasing your VO2 max means your body processes more oxygen during each breath, which makes it easier to breathe during your workout. A higher VO2 max makes exercise easier because your lungs perform more efficiently. Plus, an increase in VO2 max also lessens the volume of air you need to intake during rest. Just as your resting heart rate decreases when your heart becomes stronger, the amount of oxygen you need at rest also decreases with an increase in VO2 max. That also increases the quality of your sleep!

According to the data gathered by Firstbeat, a company that creates physiological analytics for smart wearables, here is how an increase in VO2 max impacts casually climbing a set of stairs:

> *Climbing stairs has a typical VO2 cost of 16ml/ kg/min. To walk upstairs, someone with a poor fitness level, VO2max 28, is performing at 57% of their total aerobic capacity. Meanwhile, with a VO2max of 35, those same stairs are conquered while working at only 45% capacity.* [81]

Can you imagine how much easier it feels needing only 45% of your aerobic capacity in comparison to needing 57%? *A lot easier.* This applies to all the simple daily activities you do, like walking or even standing.

Metabolic Improvements

A healthier cardiovascular system benefits your metabolism, too. Cardio exercise has been shown to produce more of the growth factor hormone FGF21,[82] which stimulates glucose uptake. Faster glucose uptake means less of a chance that glucose gets stored as fat.

A recent study in Europe concluded that "those who trained on [an] exercise bike had three times as large an increase in FGF21 production compared to those who did strength training [alone]."[83] While an increase in FGF21 won't replicate or replace the metabolic benefits of strength training, this evidence suggests that you should add at least *some* cardio to your fitness regimen.

Better Mood

Cardiovascular exercise prompts an endorphin rush that makes you feel great. It's like what Elle Woods says in the movie *Legally Blonde*:

> *Exercise gives you endorphins; endorphins make you happy and happy people just don't shoot their husbands! They just don't.*

Feeling great is… great. And a positive mood motivates you to continue reaching toward your goals.

My Story

At one point in my life, I noticed myself craving alcohol, like clockwork, every Sunday night. I wanted to drink a bottle of wine at the exact same time almost every week. I don't consider myself to have an addictive personality, and I couldn't explain these intense cravings.

Luckily, I was seeing a therapist who put two and two together…

I used to do a long run on Sunday mornings, typically 20 or more miles. After years of running 40 or more miles every week, I'd mostly quit running altogether. When the therapist realized that my routine had changed, she hypothesized that my alcohol craving was a substitute for the endorphins and dopamine that my body had grown accustomed to getting from those regular Sunday runs. Without that rush of hormones, my brain looked to alcohol to feel a similar rush.

I was addicted to running. That's not an exaggeration. I preconditioned my body for a regular weekly hormonal response, and when I stopped providing it, my body craved alcohol as a chemical substitute. Other people might have craved sweets or fats, or something even worse.

That's not a sad story; it's just an example of how powerful cardiovascular exercise can be for your brain. Like all things, balance is crucial. A little bit of cardio is good for my mood, but I don't want to be dependent on it to feel good. Neither should you.

FINAL THOUGHT

The purpose of cardio training is to improve the cardiovascular system, and cardio training is essential for optimal health. Everyone benefits from regular cardio exercise, including better sleep, better circulation, better cognitive function, better sex drive, and less risk of a heart attack. Every health and wellness program should include some form of cardiovascular exercise.

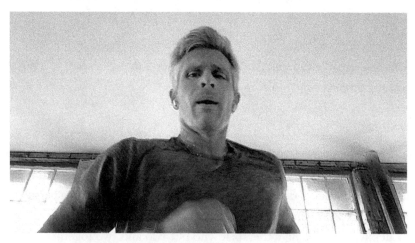

This is the face I make while struggling on a treadmill.

THE TAKEAWAY
CHAPTER 26: *THE REAL PURPOSE OF CARDIO*

The true purpose of cardio exercise is to increase the cardiovascular response.

Your heart is a muscle, and likewise, you need to train it like any other muscle in your body. Think of cardio exercise as training for your heart, and approach the training the same way you train other muscles.

Cardio exercise **increases your VO2 max** during exercise, and also results in greater cardiovascular efficiency at rest. Plus, an increase in oxygenated blood to your brain **improves cognition and decreases your risk of dementia.**

Cardio exercise **increases your metabolism** by producing more of the growth factor hormone FGF21, which increases your glucose uptake. Better glucose uptake means **less fat storage,** proving that cardio in combination with strength training can help boost your metabolism better than either on its own.

Cardio prompts your body to **release endorphins**, which improve your mood. Happy people are better equipped to achieve their goals!

CHAPTER 28

CARDIO IS NOT THE BEST WAY TO LOSE FAT

Sometimes the most difficult thing is to be able to see the most obvious thing!

MEHMET MURAT İLDAN

I previously hinted at this, but now I'm going to tell you straight-up. **Don't try to use cardio exercise to lose fat.** We've established (several times!) that to burn fat, you must be in a caloric deficit. Cardiovascular exercise indeed burns more calories than resting, but you don't actually *need* cardiovascular exercise to create a caloric deficit.

Cardio is not the solution for excess fat. Eating less food is the solution!

You may enjoy watching that calorie counter on the treadmill estimate how many calories you've burned while you jog along, staring at *CNN* on a screen hanging from the ceiling. Yes, running burns more calories per hour than walking, just like walking burns more calories per hour than sitting at your desk, and sitting at your desk burns more calories per hour than sleeping. But you don't need to burn extra calories if you don't consume them in the first place.

Another Quick Story

Coincidentally, this actually happened to me today as I was about to revise this chapter. My nanny and I were feeding my son this morning, and I asked her how she was doing. "Good! My son joined a gym and went for a nighttime workout, so the house was quiet last night." When I asked her if he liked his new gym, she said, gloomily, "I don't know. He needs to lose weight, but what he's doing doesn't make any sense."

She told me that her son went to the gym at 9 p.m. and ran on the treadmill for an hour, then he came home and ate a bag of potato chips. She's right! That approach to losing weight *doesn't make any sense.*

He went to the gym to burn calories, only to replace the calories he burned with more calories when he got home. And they weren't even nutritious calories! He ate a bunch of fat and simple carbohydrates right before bed, at a time when his body didn't need that energy. Add to that the fact that he ate poorly all day, probably consuming twice as many calories as he needed. Not only did he end the day in a caloric surplus, but he also spent an hour of his life on a treadmill, running to *nowhere.*

The Myth of Cardio as a Fat Buster

It's common for people to use cardio exercise as an excuse to eat more food than they should. People don't pay attention to how much food they eat when they assume they'll burn off those calories with cardio. They don't track their calories, they overeat, and then they do a bunch of cardio expecting everything to balance out. *It doesn't,* so they get frustrated when they don't lose weight.

But if they hadn't eaten those extra calories, then they wouldn't be in trouble. Why waste time burning calories that you didn't need to eat in the first place? That doesn't make any sense. You don't need cardio to create a caloric deficit, *you just need to eat less.*

Cardio is excellent for lots of things (see the previous chapter), but relying on cardio to create your caloric deficit is not a practical approach to fat loss. Here are a few reasons why cardio exercise is a poor way to create a caloric deficit.

Burning Calories With Cardio Takes a Long Time

You probably know people who spend hours and hours every week on the treadmill or the exercise bike, running in circles or skipping rope, climbing stairs, etc. Yes, it is possible to use cardio to create a caloric deficit. You could run on the treadmill all day, every day, thereby burning all of the calories you consume every day. But how long could you keep it up? Is that a life worth living? *No!* Cardio for the sake of burning calories is too time consuming.

I used to think I needed to run 40 miles per week to keep my weight down. I'd get up early and run five or more miles during the workweek, and then run one or two long runs of 10 to 20 miles on the weekends. I'm not a fast runner, but I've finished a dozen or so marathons and I run a 10-minute mile on average (which some people would probably consider jogging). Let's do the math on this:

10 min/mile x 40 miles/week = **400 minutes**

400 min/60 min (hour) = **6.66 hours**

I spent, on average, approximately 6.66 hours per week running. Almost one hour every day. None of that running strengthened my chest muscles, my back, my arms, or my shoulders. To train those muscles, I added strength-training workouts to my weekly routine. I'd spend about an hour in the gym, three or four times each week.

3.5 hours in gym + 6.66 hours running = **10.16 hours**

That's a lot of time for exercise in a busy schedule. And that estimate doesn't include the time I spent driving to the gym, showering, and so on. Allotting that much time to exercise won't work for most of us in the real world, with real jobs, families, and the occasional bit of fun. If that kind of exercise schedule does work for a while, it won't be sustainable in the long term.

Adult life is too hectic to spend 10 hours exercising each week! Why would you want your health to depend on having an extra 10 hours each week to spend in a gym? At some point, you won't have the time to run 40 miles a week, and the fat will come back. That's what happened to me, time and time again.

Return on Investment

Let's look at the actualized caloric benefit of all that cardio. Using an online calculator, I see that a person my weight (165 lb) running at a pace of 10 minutes/mile for 400 minutes (40 miles) burns 5,000 calories. That's 5,000 calories burned per week from cardiovascular exercise.

Sure, that's a large number of calories to add to my deficit, but is it worth the time spent exercising? Consider that I could create a similar deficit by reducing my caloric intake by 714 calories a day:

714 calories per day x 7 days = 4,998 calories (Close enough)

Cutting 714 calories is roughly equivalent to cutting the number of calories in a venti Frappuccino (470 calories[84]) and buttered croissant (260 calories[85]) from Starbucks. **How much easier would it be for you to skip the Frappuccino and the croissant than it would be to run five miles today?** You don't need to "run off" that Frappuccino... *just don't eat it!*

There are endless ways to cut 714 calories from the modern American diet. Those 714 calories could be a plate of bacon and eggs, a basket of French fries at lunch, a few extra slices of bread, or a scoop of ice cream before bed. You don't *need* to eat any of those things!

Running 40 miles a week is an extreme example, but you feel me. Statistics indicate that most of us overeat. If you've got excess fat, I can practically guarantee that you eat more calories than you need. This isn't about "dieting." *This is about being mindful of how much food your body really needs, and honoring that.* Don't use exercise as a solution to a problem that you created.

Joint Health

Many cardiovascular activities are high-impact, meaning they put excessive stress on your joints. The most popular forms of cardio (running, jogging, and biking) put a lot of pressure on your body. Your knees and hips take a beating during these activities, and doing so for extended periods of time compounds the problem.

Likewise, your ability to do high-impact cardio regularly at the levels you need to create a deficit mainly depends on your genetic predisposition to good joint health. If your knees aren't great, then it's difficult to get enough exercise to create a deficit each week. And guess what? At some point in life, *many* of us will have joint issues.

If you are reading this book, then you are most likely *not* an elite athlete. Between 65 and 80% of runners experience a joint injury every year, typically caused by overuse.[86] A running injury will wreck your fitness goals. *Why risk it?* Excessive cardio creates a high risk of injury, but there is zero risk of injury when you decide to skip the Frappuccino.

Neglecting Other Muscles

Prioritizing cardio to create a deficit may cause you to overlook other muscle groups. That leads to muscular imbalance, which may have more significant consequences than just the way you look.

If some muscles are stronger or tighter than others, you increase your risk of injury. That risk increases when the overtrained muscle is in opposition to a neglected muscle (e.g., hamstrings vs. quads). Running 40 miles a week while also sitting in a chair for eight hours each day caused my hips to lock, which eventually caused me to sprain my lower back. I spent so much time running that I didn't make time to train my legs evenly. I won't make that mistake again.

Metabolic Syndrome

I used to think I could eat whatever I wanted, *whenever* I wanted, because I was running so much. I learned the hard way that this isn't true. Monkeying with your metabolism to justify calories from junk food creates other health risks.

Using cardio to rationalize unhealthy foods—especially foods high in sugar and fat—can still lead to metabolic syndrome. You can't use that long cardio session to justify eating a pint of ice cream right before bed. The late-night binge will still disrupt your endocrine system. It isn't miraculously healthy to eat a ton of sugar before bed merely because you exercised earlier in the day.

Don't use cardio exercise as an excuse to overeat or to eat junk food. Your body doesn't work that way.

AVOID THE "FAT-BURNING" CARDIO ZONE

Cardio machines (treadmills, elliptical machines, stationary bikes, etc.) often indicate different heart rate zones for "burning fat" vs. "cardio fitness," or similar. These zones typically fall into the following ranges:

- **"Fat loss" zone:** 50–70% of max heart rate
- **Endurance zone:** 70–80% of max heart rate
- **Performance or "fitness" zone:** >80% of max heart rate or greater

I cringe when I hear trainers prescribe long-form cardio as the best way to manage weight. They suggest longer sessions (30 minutes or more) at 50 to 70% of max heart rate, three or more times per week. Sure, fat loss occurs in an aerobic state, but *what about your heart?* Long-form, steady-state cardio is not the best way to increase your cardiovascular fitness, because it doesn't push your heart hard enough to increase its strength. Your heart becomes stronger during the *anaerobic* phase of an exercise, the same way that your other muscles increase strength. To strengthen your heart muscle, you must move out of a fat-loss zone and work at greater than 80% of your maximum heart rate.

The cardio many people use to burn extra calories doesn't tax your heart enough to increase its relative strength. If you run long distances at a steady, moderate pace to burn calories, not only are you using cardio to burn calories you didn't need to eat in the first place, but you're also missing out on the *real* advantages of cardiovascular training that come from a stronger heart muscle and an increased VO2 max.

FINAL THOUGHT

Don't add cardio sessions to your program to burn extra calories. Instead, incorporate cardio exercises that strengthen your heart, and leave the extra calories on the table. If you don't eat those extra calories, you won't need to spend excessive amounts of time burning them off.

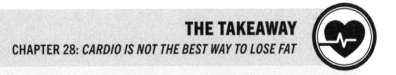

THE TAKEAWAY

CHAPTER 28: *CARDIO IS NOT THE BEST WAY TO LOSE FAT*

You don't need cardio exercise to create a caloric deficit. You can achieve a deficit by avoiding excess calories in the first place.

Using cardio to burn extra calories takes a lot of time. That's time you could spend with your family, time you could be resting, or time you could use to train your muscles. Even if you have the time now, you probably won't be that flexible for the rest of your adult life. (Unless you are super rich and single. *Congrats!*)

Excessive cardio is hard on your joints. Not everyone's body is engineered to run for an hour. Don't rely on your genetic predisposition to create a caloric deficit.

Many cardio exercises disproportionately strengthen specific muscles, and this can create muscular imbalance. Muscular imbalances lead to injury, and an injury will sabotage your fitness goals.

Don't use cardio as an excuse to eat garbage. Eating a pint of ice cream before bed still screws up your insulin response, even if you ran five miles earlier in the day. Using cardio as an excuse to justify poor eating habits can lead to metabolic dysfunction. Don't go there.

Long, slow cardio in the fat-loss zone does very little to improve your cardio-vascular fitness because it is an *aerobic* activity. The real purpose of cardio-vascular exercise is to strengthen your heart and lungs, and that happens when you work closer to your maximum heart rate.

HIIT IT!

*If everything seems under control, you're not going
fast enough.*

MARIO ANDRETTI

HIGH-INTENSITY INTERVAL TRAINING

High-intensity interval training combines short bursts of anaerobic exercise with recovery periods. It's also known as sprint interval training, or by its acronym, HIIT. Each sprint interval pushes your heart toward your maximum heart rate as quickly as possible. Ideally, you approach at least 90% of your max. You fill your lungs, and your heart beats as fast as it can to shuttle oxygenated blood to your muscles. The heart muscle works *anaerobically*, which means that it uses more ATP for harder, faster contractions.

After sprinting, you slow your heart down during a rest interval, before jumping up to high intensity again. You go back and forth like this for multiple rounds. As your heart increases in strength, it switches between these modes quicker.

You *Go! Go! Go!* really hard, and then you rest and repeat.

Exercising close to your maximum heart rate improves the strength and efficiency of your heart over time. HIIT also decreases the amount of time it takes for your heart rate to rebound after exertion. Eventually, that leads to a lower resting heart rate and, most likely, an increase in VO2 max.

Any time you spend on cardiovascular exercise should aim to improve cardiovascular fitness. As we've discussed, a stronger heart and a higher VO2 max improve metabolic function. While reaching toward your maximum heart rate might seem scary, it shouldn't be. As with any exercise, ask your doctor about your target heart rate and how far you should push yourself when sprinting.

HOW TO HIIT

My favorite type of HIIT is treadmill sprints. I find it easier to track intervals on a treadmill screen than it is to use a watch on an outdoor track. Plus, it's convenient to tack treadmill sprints on to the end of a strength-training workout because there is definitely a treadmill at your gym.

My Typical HIIT Treadmill Workout:

Two-minute warm-up at base pace

First Sprint: one-minute sprint as fast as possible

One-minute walk/jog

Second Sprint: one minute as fast as possible

One-minute walk/jog

Third Sprint: one minute as fast as possible

One-minute walk/jog

Fourth Sprint: one minute as fast as possible

One to five minutes at base pace to cool down and try not to vomit

I'm comfortable jogging at a 6 mph pace on the treadmill, so I use that as my base pace. I slow the treadmill down to a walk if that's what I need to recover. My goal is to return my heart rate to a comfortable, steady rhythm by the end of my rest interval. Once it's time to sprint again, I push myself as hard as I can for a full minute.

Over time your heart recovers faster after each sprint interval. If your heart rate returns to your resting BPM in less than 30 seconds, you should increase the speed or duration of your sprints, or decrease the duration of your rest intervals.

Classic HIIT programs often utilize shorter intervals; 40-second sprints with 20 seconds of recovery are common. However, I prefer to be in an aerobic zone during recovery intervals by maintaining my base pace, instead of walking or stopping. I bring my heart rate down, but not necessarily all the way down to my resting heart rate. Working this way increases my endurance during aerobic activities. Experiment with the duration of your HIIT intervals and figure out what works for you.

HIIT Isn't Just for the Treadmill

You can apply a high-intensity interval training pattern to almost any kind of cardio exercise. I often use the stationary bike, the ergonomic rower, or the stair climber to switch things up. Plyometric exercises also work well for HIIT rounds, and have the added benefit of increasing stability and improving functional movements. That's two or three benefits for the price of one soaked T-shirt!

But here's a warning: if you decide to try high-intensity interval training with any of these other exercises, make sure you can still increase your heart rate close to your max. If the movement is too technical and you can't repeat it quickly enough to get your heart rate up, it doesn't count as HIIT.

Some Favorite HIIT Exercises to Get You Moving:

Burpees

Battle Ropes

Mountain Climbers

Jumping Rope

Ice Skaters

Box Jumps

High Knees

Butt Kicks

Jumping Lunges

Lateral Jumps

Tuck Jumps

Star Jumps

Plank Jacks

Jumping Jacks

HOW MUCH HIIT?

"Nate, how many calories do I burn while doing HIIT? How much HIIT do I need to get ripped?"

Those are the wrong questions! The purpose of HIIT is not to burn fat. While HIIT does increase your metabolic rate at rest, you also accomplish this with strength training. Don't think about the calories you burn during a HIIT session, and please don't use the calories you burn during a HIIT session to justify eating more food!

Think of your HIIT session as another set in your strength-training regimen. You train your heart and lungs the same way you've spent the past 40 minutes training other muscles. Add a set of HIIT to the end of your strength-training workouts a few times each week. You're already at the gym, and we're talking about 10 extra minutes before you can pack up and head home. This way, you train your heart and lungs as part of your total fitness program.

I pick HIIT exercises that *complement* the muscles I'm training that day. On a leg day, I try the exercise bike or the ergonomic rower. If I trained my arms, I'd do a few HIIT sets of battle ropes.

Experiment with what works for you, but don't overtrain. If it's a rest day for a specific muscle because you worked it yesterday, don't push that muscle with HIIT today. Likewise, if you worked your arms to exhaustion today, skip the battle ropes and jump on the treadmill. If you can't push yourself toward your maximum heart rate because your muscles are Jell-O from lifting, try a different HIIT exercise.

THE TAKEAWAY
CHAPTER 29: *HIIT IT!*

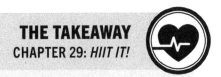

Use High-intensity interval training to train your heart like every other muscle in your body. It improves cardiovascular fitness and you can finish an effective HIIT workout in 10 minutes. No more spending hours on the treadmill!

» HIIT is composed of sprint intervals at, or close to, your maximum heart rate and short recovery intervals to bring your heart back to its resting BPM.

» You can do HIIT with many different types of exercises, but get your heart rate above 80% of its maximum during the sprint intervals, or it doesn't count as HIIT.

Pick HIIT exercises that complement your strength-training schedule, and consider tacking them on to the end of your strength-training workout. Be sure to honor rest days that are part of your training program, and don't overtrain muscles with HIIT.

WALK IT OFF

If your dog is fat, you're not getting enough exercise.

UNKNOWN

I've been wearing one fitness tracker or another for over five years. Why? Because they help motivate me to keep *walking*. I walk an average of 12,000 steps a day. That's approximately four miles. Sometimes I walk more than that, like when I'm on vacation or if I'm competing in the app with friends who want to push their step goal. Regardless, I try not to let that number fall below 10,000 steps each day.

Based on my stats, walking four miles at a slowish, comfortable pace takes me about an hour and 30 minutes and burns approximately 370 calories. That's about the same number of calories I'd burn if I were jogging at a pace of 5.5 mph for 30 minutes, but the time I spend walking is split up throughout the day. I rack up steps when I walk to the grocery store, the mailbox, or just to the living room.

Walking these steps makes a massive difference in my life in many ways, not just in the total number of calories I burn. I don't think of walking as added exercise; I think of it as part of my lifestyle. Here are the reasons I choose to walk instead of jogging every day.

I Don't Need to Schedule Time to Walk

I don't get sweaty when I walk for 10 minutes on my lunch break. Unlike running I can walk intermittently throughout the day without needing to shower and change my clothes. I walk my dogs twice a day, I walk to the post office, and I take a long walk with my family after dinner. I spend a little extra time walking instead of driving. Walking passively increases my caloric deficit without monopolizing my time like dedicated exercise does. Plus, the fresh air breaks up my workday.

Walking Doesn't Zap My Energy

Running or jogging tires me out quickly. That means timing food around the run. If I eat beforehand, I get bloated while exercising. If I wait to eat too long afterward, I go into starvation mode (i.e., I get *hangry*). But walking is much easier on my body. I can walk with a full stomach, and I can also walk a long stretch without getting ravenous afterward. Walking works all the time, regardless of my "feeding" schedule.

Walking Doesn't Stress My Joints

Running and jogging can be murder on your knees, and the problem worsens if you are out of shape or very muscular. (More weight means more stress on your joints, even if the weight is muscle mass.) Walking is low-impact and keeps your body accustomed to moving the way it was designed to move.

Walking Reduces Stress

This might be the biggest benefit to walking. Regular walking has been shown to reduce levels of cortisol (the stress hormone), in particular when those walks happen outside in natural settings.[87] Less stress means more strength to accomplish your goals!

WALK MORE

Make a plan to get up and walk for a few minutes at various times throughout the day. I set an alarm* to remind me to move at least 250 steps each hour, because long stretches of sitting at my desk are torturous on my back. The alarm gets me off my butt. Breaking my day up with walks forces me to flex my hips and hamstrings and increases my step count.

Consider a similar strategy, especially if you work in an office. You might take a stroll to check in on a colleague, walk around the floor of your building, or step outside for a minute of fresh air. You'll increase your total daily energy expenditure and ensure your future mobility.

---

* Fitness trackers like Fitbit, Apple Watch, etc. include alarms for this purpose.

THE TAKEAWAY
CHAPTER 30: *WALK IT OFF*

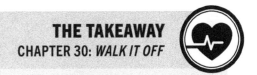

Walking is a convenient way to increase your TDEE. It also improves circulation and may prevent back pain caused by sitting for extended periods.

Find opportunities to walk throughout your day. Walk to the store, the post office, whatever. It's a small investment of time that will reward you in many ways.

Set an alarm or create a regular reminder to get up and walk for five to 10 minutes of every hour during the workday.

PART FIVE

OTHER CONSIDERATIONS

THE ONLY FITNESS SUPPLEMENTS I USE

A shortcut is the longest distance between two points.

CHARLES ISSAWI

HOW DO I CHOOSE FITNESS SUPPLEMENTS?

I'm very selective about the nutritional supplements I take. If I feel like finding a new fitness supplement—*because, why not?*—I visit my local GNC store, and I look for the bottle with the shiniest wrapper. You know the one. It reads, "FAT X-PLODE!!" in hot pink letters, and there's a photo of a man on the label with minus-2% body fat. I will spend my last 50 dollars on that bottle if the person behind the counter promises me that the 2,000 grams of caffeine in this pill definitely won't cause me to shake violently when I try to fall asleep at night. I believe him! HE WORKS HERE!

That's a joke. I'm kidding, of course.

Unfortunately, many people try fitness supplements based on similar strategies. They just pick something up and hope it changes their life. Unfortunately, there's an entire industry built around false promises (read: lies) about pills that create instantaneous fat loss or miraculous muscle gain, and many people fall for it.

Don't believe the lies! Pills won't "melt" fat off your body like some kind of laser gun. You can take all the fitness supplements in the world, but if you eat more calories than you burn, you will still hold on to the fat. Then you'll be fat *and* jittery.

Six Supplements to Consider

There are only six fitness supplements you should consider at this point:

- BCAAs;
- Whey protein powder;
- Carbohydrate powder;
- Creatine;
- Vitamins and Minerals; and
- Casein.

These are the supplements I use to augment my strength-training regimen and to help balance my macronutrient ratios. They aren't required for fat loss or muscle gain, and they certainly won't do either of those things on their own. They are *supplements*, which means they are intended to supplement a diet and exercise program that includes a caloric deficit.

This list of six might seem long or intimidating if you are new to all of this. Please know that I've put a lot of time and *personal research* into using them. (I didn't just pull a list from a fitness magazine.) But remember that you don't *need* these supplements to achieve your goals. They are merely what I use to supplement my current eating habits and lifestyle, and I'm confident that you can achieve similar results without them. Don't stress if they are too expensive or if they give you gas! Just skip 'em.

Here they are, in order of when I take them throughout the day:

BCAA

What Is It?

Branched-chain amino acids.

When Do I Use It?

Just before or during my workout.

Why Do I Use It?

I prefer to work out first thing (or second thing) in the morning. Some people feel like they need carbohydrates to get them moving in the morning, but I don't like to eat before I lift. I feel sluggish and bloated if I eat a meal before exercising, especially if I'm doing cardio. All I need is coffee and, occasionally, a handful of dried apricots.

Since I train in a fasted state, I use a BCAA supplement during my workout. BCAAs are the building blocks of protein, the stuff that makes up muscle mass. The three branched-chain amino acids are leucine, isoleucine, and valine. These are three of the nine essential amino acids required by our bodies.

You wake up in the morning in a fasted state (unless you're a person who raids the fridge in the middle of the night). It's as if you've been on a mini-diet for the last six to nine hours. As I've mentioned before, if your body needs energy but doesn't have any food to digest, it begins to look elsewhere for that energy. If you lift weights in a fasted state, there is a chance that your body will begin to catabolize muscle tissue to free amino acids it can use for fuel.

That's a problem. Muscle catabolism is one of the reasons people often lose muscle mass while dieting. BCAA supplements are useful in this scenario, because they balance against the loss of amino acids from muscle catabolism. Ingesting leucine especially has been proven to increase protein synthesis,[88,89,90] adding another weapon against protein breakdown while exercising in a fasted state. Plus, drinking a BCAA mixture keeps you hydrated during a workout because it's mostly water.

How Important Is a BCAA Supplement?

We can, theoretically, get all the amino acids we need from food. But there is a catch: food must be *digested* to release those amino acids into your system. Digestion is a function I want to avoid while I'm exercising. I don't want to walk around the gym with a gut full of whey protein powder or anything else. A belly full of food will weigh me down or, worse, make me farty. *No thanks!*

However, a BCAA supplement is a powder that contains zero calories, not a food. As such, adding some to my water before a workout does not make me feel bloated or uncomfortable. Instead, it simply prepares me for the work I plan to do.

One Note of Caution:

Some commercial BCAA mixtures also include caffeine, nitric oxide boosters, etc. You don't want any of that stuff. Check the label carefully on any "pre-workout" supplement, and follow the recommended dosage. If you experience any side effects, check with a physician.

WHEY PROTEIN POWDER

What Is It?

The liquid that forms when milk is curdled (separated). It is a complete protein containing all nine essential amino acids and is low in lactose.

When Do I Use It?

Immediately after my workout.

Why Do I Use It?

The body needs protein after a workout to prevent muscle catabolism and to begin the muscle-building process. Whey protein is the fastest, most efficient way to consume protein after training. It is easier to digest than other forms of protein, such as casein or a chicken breast.

"But Nate," you ask, "didn't you drink a BCAA mixture? Doesn't this do the same thing?" Good question! But no, it doesn't. Unlike a BCAA powder, whey protein is a *complete* protein. It contains all nine essential amino acids, not just the three branched-chain amino acids.

Some people argue against the importance of ingesting protein immediately after a workout, and research exists to support both opinions. Your total daily protein intake is much more critical than *when* you consume it. I'm merely stating what works for me, and I've had great results by sucking down a protein shake after I lift. Do what works for you!

I try to do everything I can to support the muscle mass I have while trying to lose fat. I don't want my body pulling energy from my muscles. A protein shake tells my body to immediately begin building muscle as a response to the physical stress I've just endured. I aim to convince my metabolism that we are in a building phase, even when I'm trying to lose fat.

It's also easy to drink a shake after my workout. *Convenience, baby!*

How Do I Choose a Whey Protein?

I typically use a filtered, lactose-free whey protein powder because lactose makes me gassy. However, I recently tried a brand that doesn't specifically advertise itself to be lactose-free and I love the taste. I haven't experienced any adverse reactions so I'm sticking with it for now. (Ping me if you are interested in the details, or check out the brands I recommend at fitnrd. com/stuff.) I suggest balancing taste against nutritional composition. Also, be sure to check how much sugar or other carbohydrate is in the formula.

If you don't like the taste of whey or find that it argues with your insides, there are many substitute protein powders on the market now. These include products made from beef, egg whites, and various plant proteins. Look for a complete protein source, and try a few options until you land on something you can stomach.

CARBOHYDRATE POWDER

What Is It?

A powder consisting solely of high-glycemic carbohydrates (i.e., a simple sugar in powdered form).

When Do I Use It?

Immediately after my workout.

Why Do I Use It?

Here's where my post-workout shake gets interesting. You've probably heard of whey protein powder, but did you know that carbohydrates also come in powder form? These are often straight dextrose or maltodextrin—two simple sugars that metabolize rapidly. I mix one of these powders directly into my whey protein shake so that I can drink both supplements at the same time.

Yes, I add sugar to my protein shake. Does that blow your mind?

A few years ago, if anyone had told me, "Nate, you need to consume a bunch of high-GI carbs right after your workout," I would have done a spit-take with my protein shake. I've seen high-calorie mass building supplements at the health food store, but I've always ignored them because I was taught to cut carbs when I wanted to lean out. Now I know that limiting carbohydrates on training days was inhibiting my ability to gain muscle mass.

The Sugar Rush

Your body uses most of the glucose in your system during a workout. If you lift in a fasted state, that amount of glucose is already quite low. Additionally, you probably dipped into some of the glycogen stored in your muscles as an additional energy source. After your workout, your blood sugar is presumably lower than its baseline.

You need to restore glucose and glycogen stores after a workout so that your body doesn't trigger the starvation response. You can replace glucose and glycogen rapidly by consuming high-GI carbohydrate powder immediately post-exercise. Having a small amount of simple carbohydrates right then will bring you back to your baseline blood sugar level.

This is especially crucial for any high-intensity interval training where fast-twitch muscles are taxed. Have you ever heard of Gatorade? *That is why drinks like that exist!*

Consuming a high-GI carbohydrate provokes the insulin response because insulin is the hormone your body uses to regulate glucose as an energy source. Post-workout is precisely the right time for insulin.

"So, can I eat a Snickers bar after my workout, brah?"

No. Absolutely not, brah. You are still trying to stay lean. That means avoiding refined sugars most of the time, and always avoiding high-fructose corn syrup and the like. However, consuming a controlled portion of natural sugar immediately after a workout can benefit muscle growth.

Which Carb Powder Should You Use?

Don't get bogged down by fake science that tells you one brand of carb powder enters your bloodstream 10 seconds faster than another. That's marketing bullshit. There are competing philosophies about the post-workout benefits of dextrose (a monosaccharide) versus maltodextrin (a slightly more complex carbohydrate, or "starch"). But both do the same thing within a sufficient time frame, so your choice depends on how your body responds to each of these simple carbs.

I prioritize taste, convenience, and cost when I shop for a carb powder. Here's what I'm looking for:

- Must be flavorless, because I add it to whey protein (I don't want to drink two separate shakes at once)
- Must be easy to mix, meaning it dissolves easily
- Must have limited or no fructose
- Must be caffeine-free, because I don't want any more caffeine after a workout
- Must be free of additional protein and dairy because I get protein from the whey
- Only carbohydrates—nothing else

Carb Powder Brands I Like (As of December 2019):

It's not always easy to find a supplement that meets my requirements. Most post-workout carbohydrate supplements come premixed with protein, etc., or they come in the form of a fruity powder that doesn't taste good when mixed with chocolate whey powder. Unlike elsewhere, I've listed actual brands here because carb powders can be harder to come by. Again, check fitnrd.com/stuff for links to the brands I currently use.

- **Waxy Maize.** Very similar to corn starch (maltodextrin). Claims of super-quick absorption are a bit overkill, but this product does what I need it to do, and it adheres to the six requirements above.
- **Universal Nutrition Carbo Plus.** This is primarily a malto-dextrin supplement, and it's made by a reputable company that's been around for a long time.
- **Performix Carbon.** A dextrose supplement. Dextrose is an even simpler sugar than maltodextrin, and Carbon tastes very sweet, like table sugar. It might be discontinued by the time you read this, but I've included it because it's what I currently use. As of December 2019, it is still available from Performix via Amazon.

How Important Is a Carb Powder?

Adding sugar to my protein shake has made a huge difference for me. I've noticed that I'm better able to regulate my blood sugar throughout the day if I use one of these powders after I lift. It prevents my blood sugar from dropping too low mid-morning, so I don't get *hangry*. Also, it may be coincidental, but I was able to add lean muscle while maintaining a deficit, and I do attribute this in part to adding carb powders to my planning.

If you hope to maintain muscle while losing fat—or to build muscle during a bulking phase—try a carb powder. Just remember to drink it immediately after your workout and in conjunction with your target daily macronutrient balance. Don't consume high-GI foods in times of inactivity, or you risk storing those calories as fat. No, you can't throw carb powder in your iced tea at dinner!

> **SIDE NOTE:** There are other ways besides powders to get a jolt of high-glycemic carbohydrates post-workout. I often eat an apple after I lift, which adds fructose to the mix. The apple includes a little fiber and keeps me feeling full until I eat a real meal (about one hour after my workout). Immediately post-workout is typically the only time I eat simple carbs all day (all other carbs will be complex), so I enjoy fruit during this window.

CREATINE

What Is It?

Creatine is a nonessential nutrient created by the body to facilitate ATP transportation into cells.

When Do I Use It?

Immediately after my workout. (Yes, I add it to the whey protein and carb powder shake.)

Why Do I Use It?

Earlier, I briefly explained how our cells use adenosine triphosphate (ATP) for energy at the cellular level. After an ATP molecule gives up a phosphate to create energy, it becomes adenosine *di*phosphate (ADP).

Creatine binds with phosphate to become *creatine-phosphate* and then shuttles that extra phosphate back to the ADP; this in turn converts that molecule back into ATP. In theory, a creatine supplement increases the amount of ATP at our disposal. Our muscle cells then have the energy they need from ATP instead of relying on glycogen stores or catabolizing muscle tissue for energy. That's the gist.

Do I Need It?

There is evidence to show that supplementing creatine to create a creatine surplus aids in ATP storage and therefore makes more energy available during strenuous exercise.[91, 92] We get normal levels of creatine from food and our bodies produce some creatine naturally, but we can only store a small amount of it as a reserve. This is why some professionals advocate loading creatine by taking large doses (>15 g) every day for a few days to increase the amount stored in their bodies for times of greater expenditure (e.g., when strength training).

Many bodybuilders supplement their creatine intake with commercial products. Vegetarians commonly supplement creatine, because humans get most of our creatine from meat.

Is Creatine Safe?

Creatine is a well-studied supplement and is generally recognized as low-risk.[93] The European Food Safety Administration released a statement in 2004 stating that creatine supplementation of up to three grams per day is safe.[94]

Many people load with much more creatine than this, but I believe that's pointless. As I mentioned, there is a limit to how much creatine your body can store, and excess creatine is mostly filtered out of your body through the liver and kidneys. That may lead to kidney failure or liver toxicity in people at higher risk of those issues. Research shows that regular creatine use by healthy athletes doesn't negatively impact renal function,[95] but why risk it by surpassing the recommended dose?

How Much Do I Take and When?

I take a maintenance dose of five grams per day to make sure there is enough creatine in my system without putting undue stress on my kidneys or liver. It's the last ingredient I add to my post-workout protein shake. I supplement with five grams of post-workout creatine for three weeks out of the month, and then I abstain for a week to allow my body's natural equilibrium to reset, ensuring that I still produce normal levels of creatine on my own.

How to Choose a Creatine Supplement

You want the purest creatine you can get, but it isn't worth spending a fortune on "super-duper micro-ionized triple-filter *blah-blah*." That's marketing hype.

I look for creatine supplements that are flavorless and don't contain any extra stuff, like sugar, fake sugar, or caffeine. I add it to the whey protein and the carbo powder, so I need it all to taste good together.

VITAMINS & MINERALS

What Are Vitamins and Minerals?

Are you kidding me? Okay, sure, I'll tell you. These are small organic (vitamins) and inorganic (minerals) compounds required by the body to function.

When Do I Use Them?

Lunchtime!

Why Do I Use Them?

I take a vitamin and mineral supplement every day. Yes, you can indeed get all the vitamins and minerals you need from a balanced diet. The same goes for protein, sugar, and creatine.

However, the balance of vitamins and minerals in the body fluctuates based on diet, and diet is contingent on the time of year because different foods are available during different seasons. I'm lucky to live in Los Angeles, and I can usually get tomatoes anytime I want them. But sometimes during colder months they taste like garbage or they are imported from places with authoritarian governments that I don't support (*sorry, not sorry*), so I avoid them.

Additionally, some vitamins are dependent upon external sources. For example, a certain form of vitamin D (vitamin D3) is only produced by the body when the skin is exposed to sunlight. During short winter days when my sun exposure is low, I don't produce enough vitamin D.

I supplement vitamin intake with an Animal Pak. I take one pack every day. It's not so much that I risk an overdose, but it's enough to be an insurance policy against slips in my diet. I take the regular Animal Pak—not a "sterol stack" or any of the other supplements they offer now. It's basically the same Animal Pak my dad has taken for 30 years. I know the company behind it, Universal Nutrition, maintains the high quality and consistency of their product and has been doing so for decades.

You might also consider a multivitamin. Talk to your doctor if you have any questions or feel like you may have a vitamin deficiency.

Are Vitamin and Mineral Supplements Crucial?

Nope. I take vitamins and minerals in small doses as a matter of general wellness. Unless a doctor has identified a deficiency in your diet, you are probably fine. Have blood work done if you're suspicious.

CASEIN

What Is It?

Casein is the other protein in dairy. (Whey being the first.)

When Do I Use It?

Nighttime, before bed.

Why Do I Use It?

Casein is a milk-based protein that digests much more slowly than whey. It is also naturally lactose-free. I take a casein shake before bed so that the protein digests in my system overnight. This provides a small amount of protein to my bloodstream while I sleep.

Nighttime is when I would otherwise be in a "fasted" state. I'm sleeping, so that's seven or more hours without eating. The night is also the time when my body runs its maintenance and housekeeping cycles, and that includes muscle building! I supplement with casein so that I have protein in my system to fuel that muscle building for at least part of the night.

I know serious lifters (like my former roommate) who would set the alarm in the middle of the night to wake up and eat more protein. I'm not going to do that because I'm prone to acid reflux if I lay down with a full stomach of food. A casein shake before bed hasn't given me any tummy trouble so far (knock on wood), so it's a nice compromise.

I'll also often eat a small portion of fat (typically 0.5 ounces of raw almonds) with the casein to help prevent the starvation response.

As with any food you ingest before bed, exercise caution, and talk to your doctor if you have concerns. Acid reflux is dangerous, for real, so it's best not to eat any solid foods for at least an hour before you lay down.

* * *

A WARNING ABOUT FAT-BURNING SUPPLEMENTS

Fat burners are typically stimulants or diuretics, often including high doses of caffeine.* They screw with your energy, your blood pressure, your endocrine system, and more, and as a result, they can be very dangerous. (Remember Fen-Phen, anyone?) Any weight loss you may experience is most likely water loss, or the starvation response causes it.

Be afraid of "fat-burning" supplements. I've tried many varieties of fat burners in my quest to lose weight. (Yeah, I'm guilty of trying to cheat the math, too.) I suggest you avoid any pill that claims to aid in fat loss. Remember, there are no shortcuts... other than liposuction.

Fat burners are only suitable for professional lifters who already have very low body fat. They use them sparingly when preparing for a contest or a photo shoot because they want to be dehydrated. The effects are temporary, and they aren't worth the risks.

---

* I consider caffeine to be a drug, not a fitness supplement, although some people use it that way. Caffeine has many positive and negative effects on the body, and its complexity is beyond the scope of this book. Talk to your doctor to determine safe levels of caffeine intake based on your current health.

Earlier this year, I accidentally tried a fat burner that was included in a vitamin supplement I tried. *I didn't sleep for three days.* So, heed my advice and **avoid fat burners.** Maintain a caloric deficit, and you will lose fat without feeling like you're amped on 10 gallons of coffee.

FAKE SUGARS IN SUPPLEMENTS (A DISCLAIMER)

Some of the supplements I take include fake sugars or chemical sweeteners. If you've read this book, you know I mostly avoid those things. However, I typically use the supplements listed here early in the day—in coordination with a workout—in a way that allows me to control my insulin response. I find that the positives (convenience and macro-impact) outweigh the negatives (some fake sugar and chemicals). Still, you should test them out and see if they work for you. If something doesn't feel right in any way, stop using it!

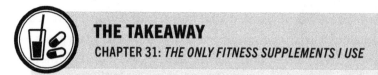

THE TAKEAWAY

CHAPTER 31: *THE ONLY FITNESS SUPPLEMENTS I USE*

Fitness supplements are not required for fat loss. They are a boost to help you achieve the results you are after, mainly by offering you convenience. They aren't necessary.

The supplements I use are:

» BCAA powder;

» Whey protein powder;

» A high-GI carbohydrate powder;

» Creatine;

» A vitamin and mineral supplement; and

» Casein. *That's it.*

These are the only supplements I take consistently, and I use them in conjunction with a well-balanced, mostly clean diet. In my opinion, most other supplements are either (a) dangerous or (b) a waste of time.

Avoid fat burners! Don't take any supplement that claims to accelerate fat loss. They are dangerous, and they aren't a substitute for a caloric deficit.

CHAPTER 32

GO THE FUCK TO SLEEP

I know you're not thirsty.
That's bullshit. Stop lying.
Lie the fuck down, my darling, and sleep.

ADAM MANSBACH, *Go the Fuck to Sleep*

THE EFFECTS OF SLEEP DEPRIVATION

I've never been great about getting enough sleep. Then I had a baby and getting a good night's sleep became nearly impossible. I love my kid to the moon and back, but I was averaging less than four hours a night for almost a year after he was born. If you have kids, you know this challenge and you know sleep deprivation *sucks*.

I'm amazed by how much the quality of our sleep impacts daily life. It influences our mood, our ability to concentrate at work, our energy levels, and how much crap we can tolerate from those around us. And in addition to the myriad mental, emotional, and social ramifications of sleep loss, there are devastating physiological and biochemical consequences to a lack of zzz's. Chronic sleep deficiency leads to an increased risk of heart disease, high blood pressure, kidney disease, diabetes, and more.[96] That's because your body runs its "maintenance" cycles while you sleep. It's the time of peak hormone release, facilitating cellular repair and reproduction.

Without sleep, you die. *Harsh, but true.*

Sleep and Hormones

Sleep also plays a vital physiological role in any fat-loss program by regulating the hormones that govern your appetite. There is a reason you get hungry when you're tired! Sleep allows the body to balance leptin, the hormone that makes you feel satiated or "full," with ghrelin, the hormone that drives hunger. When you're sleep-deprived, your leptin levels decrease, and your ghrelin levels increase. That might be why you're guzzling that Pumpkin Spice Latte and inhaling that scone so quickly in the morning.

A study at the University of Chicago found that the quantity of sleep has a profound effect on fat loss. A group of volunteers was observed during two 14-week fat-loss programs, with each round incorporating the same caloric deficit and activity levels. Each individual was restricted to consume only 90% of the calories required to maintain their weight (i.e., a 10% caloric deficit from their TDEE), without additional exercise.

During the first 14-week period, the participants stayed in bed for 8.5 hours and slept approximately seven hours and 25 minutes on average. At the end of the round, each person lost an average of 3.1 pounds of fat mass and 3.3 pounds of lean mass (muscle).

During the second 14-week period, the participants engaged in the same caloric deficit—10%—and the same daily activities. However, their sleep was restricted to 5.5 hours in bed, resulting in an average of five hours and 14 minutes of sleep. At the end of the second 14-week round, the participants had lost an average of 1.3 pounds of fat and 5.3 lb of lean mass (muscle).[97]

Holy smokes. Not only did higher levels of ghrelin—the hungry hormone—increase appetite and reduce energy expenditure, the research also shows that lack of sleep promotes fat retention and leads to muscle catabolization. If you're struggling to achieve fat loss despite the accuracy of your deficit calculations, a lack of sleep might be the culprit.

Sleep and Insulin

When you don't get enough sleep, there is a higher than usual probability that your body won't process sugar the way it should. This idea mimics what I've said about the starvation response: if your body thinks there is a shortage of food, then it will naturally fight to conserve energy *at all costs*. Fat in your body is a long-term energy source, and it's less metabolically active than muscle. That means your body favors it in times of crisis. It's a more significant source of energy, while also not requiring as much energy as lean tissues, so naturally your body clings to it.

According to the National Heart, Lung, and Blood Institute, "sleep deficiency results in a higher than normal blood sugar level."[98] There may be a correlation between lack of sleep and insulin resistance. Research by the Endocrinology and Metabolism Clinics of North America associated sleep apnea with impaired glucose intolerance. Whether the apnea was caused by obesity or vice versa, it's clear that "the quality and quantity of sleep may have a profound effect on obesity and type 2 diabetes."[99]

Think of sleep deprivation the same way you think of the starvation response—after all, you're starving your body of rest. It's not just about how fast your metabolism works under duress. It also involves multiple other factors that contribute to how varied physiological processes coordinate with each other for your survival. Cumulatively, these processes add up to determine whether you lose fat, muscle, or neither.

HOW MUCH SLEEP IS ENOUGH?

I suggest that you get at least seven to eight hours of sleep each night. When I get less sleep than that—*like now, while editing this book*—I notice a significant slowdown in fat loss, regardless of the consistency of my caloric deficit. But this amount doesn't include the time you spend tossing and turning. For many of us, seven hours of sleep means eight to nine hours in bed.

The exact amount of sleep you need depends on each individual, within limits. You may believe that you only need four hours of sleep each night, but most doctors and scientists disagree. The bottom line: don't sabotage your goals by staying up late to watch *Game of Thrones* on demand again. *Go the fuck to sleep!*

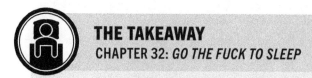

THE TAKEAWAY
CHAPTER 32: *GO THE FUCK TO SLEEP*

You need to sleep to regulate the hormones that govern your metabolism. A lack of sleep likely results in losing muscle mass instead of fat when maintaining a caloric deficit. Sleep is crucial for building the body of your dreams.

Poor sleeping habits may cause insulin resistance. Research shows a correlation between sleep deprivation and metabolic dysfunction, including glucose intolerance.

Lack of sleep results in lower energy and affects your emotions. Losing fat is already hard enough. Why complicate things by putting yourself in a bad mood?

The average adult needs a minimum of seven to eight hours of sleep each night. That number doesn't include the time you lay in bed watching television, or the time you spend tossing and turning while your partner snores like a bear.

If you're serious about losing fat and gaining lean muscle, shut your phone off and **go the fuck to sleep.**

GROUP FITNESS

I'm not in this world to live up to your expectations
and you're not in this world to live up to mine.

BRUCE LEE

SHOULD YOU TAKE THAT
"THAI-ZUMBA-P90-XTREME-CARDIO-YOGA-BARRE CLASS?"

I have a friend who takes that class. He wears a heart monitor during the workout. He and his classmates compete to see who can make their heart explode first. There's a flat-screen TV with a leaderboard that broadcasts everyone's heart rate, so my middle-aged friend can compare himself to the 19-year-old next to him. *As if he couldn't take one look at that twink and know that he's going to lose this battle.*

That craziness is not for me—hard pass. But, you do you.

I won't tell you not to take that Thai-Zumba-P90-Xtreme-Cardio-Yoga-Barre class if it works for you. Everyone needs to exercise, and you gotta do what you gotta do to keep moving. If you enjoy those classes, then go for it! Group fitness classes work for lots of people.

Some people like the camaraderie. *Don't talk to me because I am trying not to trip on this treadmill.*

Other people like the techno music they play in class. *I think the music sounds like aliens are attacking me from the sky.*

Some people want a pushy fitness instructor. *I want that guy to piss off.*

If you *need* to take classes to get your butt in gear, I feel ya. But if you are looking to try something *new*, here are a few things to keep in mind before you commit to that class pack.

A Little Competition Goes a Long Way

Peer pressure is powerful. The herd mentality favors bigger, faster, harder over safety and technique. Competitive exercise classes only benefit you when you know what you're doing.

That's especially true for classes that incorporate resistance training. I've mentioned CrossFit, but there are also many other boot camp workout classes gaining popularity. These classes have you sprint on a treadmill one minute, only to then run across the room and do dumbbell presses on a "bench" that was designed for step aerobics. With 30 people in the room, it's difficult for an instructor to make sure you're doing it all correctly.

It's hard to feel good when the guy next to you is doing shoulder presses with 25 pounds in each hand, and you're holding the little pink five-pounders because that's where you are today. It's even harder when the teacher keeps barking at you to bump up the weight.

Sometimes you will be the slowest, weakest, newest person in a group fitness class. We have all been that person at one time or another, and we will all be there again. It's tough to fight the feeling of inadequacy when you fall behind the group. That's human instinct.

But feeling inadequate is a fast track toward self-sabotage and abandoning your goals.

When I'm in a class setting, I tend to forget that everyone is different. We all have different bodies and different goals for those bodies. Comparing my performance to others is distracting me from my path. I don't need any more distractions in life.

Instead, I compete against myself. I'm here to challenge myself to do better. To beat my previous best. To go an extra 10 seconds without collapsing. I am my own competition.

The "group" in "group fitness" can be a positive motivator in the right situations, but for me, it's usually more of a distraction than it is a valuable tool. If you're in a group, make sure you put yourself and your goals ahead of any expectations from the class or instructor. Listen to your body, practice good form at a speed that feels safe to you, and if you find yourself sacrificing either of those things, skip the class.

Schedules May Vary

Are you sure those classes are convenient for your schedule? Check out the times and plan before committing to a class pack or program.

I prefer to exercise on my schedule when it's convenient for me. That might mean 6 a.m. one day, and 9 p.m. another day.

If I sleep in and don't get to the gym until 6:05 a.m., I still get the same workout I was going to get at six. Nobody is going to lock the door and tell me I'm too late for my workout.

If your training program relies on classes, then you are beholden to someone else's schedule. It's too easy to skip a class because you are running five minutes late and have back-to-back meetings ahead of you for the rest of the day.

For example, there is one popular fitness class near me that I take on occasion. The classes are fun, and the instructors are attentive. So, earlier this year, I bought a class pack, assuming I'd take a class once a week to mix things up.

I went to a class in January, but I didn't go back for four months because there never seemed to be a class that worked with my schedule. Guess what? The class credits I purchased expired, and those assholes kept my money. *Ugh*.

Classes Are Expensive

Maybe money is no object for you, but that's not the case for most of us.

The more expensive your exercise program is, **the more likely you are to drop it when your budget tightens**. Why risk it?

Single classes in LA cost $20 per class on average. That means $100/week if you exercise five times each week. That's $400/month. They convolute this price with packs and bundles and the occasional deal, but it still costs a lot to work out a few times every week.

However, most gyms near me charge between $30 and $80 a month for a membership that you can use whenever you want, as many times as you want. Even the fancy gym with the eucalyptus towels is *less than half the cost* of a month's worth of group fitness classes.

Keep your workout strategy affordable and straightforward so you never find yourself cutting exercise out of your monthly budget.

FINAL THOUGHT

Group fitness classes work for people who struggle to motivate on their own. But exercise classes are riddled by distractions. If you are human (hint: you are!), you can and will be distracted by other people, schedules that don't fit your own, and financial concerns. This doesn't even account for the instructor playing that song you hate* while you are in the middle of a grueling set of pull-ups. That shit definitely happens.

Why risk it? Find the motivation you need from within. You won't be reliant on someone else to motivate you, or dependent on class availability or a hefty bank account. I suggest a self-directed weight-training program to get the results you want, not the results the instructor, your friend, or the 19-year-old twink across the room wants.

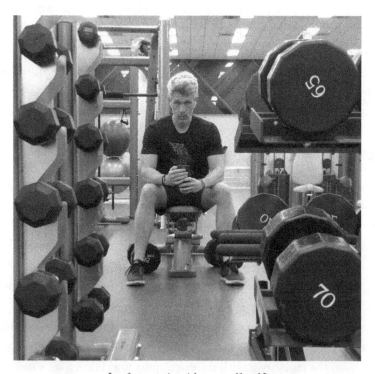

I prefer to exercise with me, myself, and I.

---

* For me, this song is Britney Spears' "...Baby One More Time." *No, thanks!* Let's leave 1999 where it belongs.

THE TAKEAWAY
CHAPTER 33: *GROUP FITNESS*

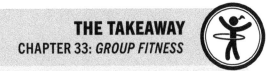

Classes foster competition (and sometimes jealousy), which may distract you from your own goals or, worse, proper form.

Classes happen on their schedule, not yours. Don't rely on someone else's schedule to get your work done.

Classes are expensive in comparison to a regular gym membership. Don't let money stand in the way of your fitness goals!

Learning what to do in a gym, on your own, will benefit you more than merely waiting for someone else to tell you what to do.

CHAPTER 34

GYM PET PEEVES

Rudeness is the weak man's imitation of strength.[*]

EDMUND BURKE

I couldn't write about strength training without mentioning the random things gym-goers do to piss me off. I probably sound like a cranky old fart yelling at the kids to "get off my lawn," but there are a few basic manners everyone should follow in the gym. Most of these things are common sense, and some of them fall into the category of treating people well *outside* of the gym, too. Please remember that you are not the only person who works out at this gym. You need to respect your fellow gym-goers, the facility, and the employees.

Still, some people are jerks, and I see these shenanigans all the time. So here we go...

MY LIST OF <u>DON'T'S</u> AND <u>DO'S</u> AT THE GYM

DON'T forget to rerack your weights when you finish an exercise.

There is only one leg press machine at my gym. Fifty percent of the time, I walk over to use it and discover that some jerk has left 10 45-pound plates on it. Five plates on each side! WTF?! Yes, I could waste my time removing all the plates you were too lazy to remove, but what about the 70-year-old

---

[*] Yes, I've quoted Edmund Burke. But this is not a political book, so please don't @ me.

woman next to me who is also here to work on her fitness? It might take her 20 minutes to clean up the 450 pounds you left out. PUT YOUR SHIT AWAY. Please be courteous and rerack your weights in the correct place. This is a skill we all learned in kindergarten, and it applies in the gym too.

DO wipe your puddle of sweat off that bench or machine.

Nobody wants to sit down in a pool of your slime, especially not in the age of COVID-19. *Come on!* Most gyms provide hand towels now. If yours doesn't, then it's *your* responsibility to bring your own or find a paper towel to wipe that shit up. Don't be a pig.

DO be conscientious of your time on a machine or bench.

If you use an app (like I do) to track your rest time, you know exactly how long you are holding up a machine in between sets. When your rest time exceeds a minute and a half, it'd be kind of you to offer for someone else to "work in." How do you know when someone is waiting for the machine you are using? Use context clues: they've been working on all the same chest machines as you for the last three exercises, and now you are on the only cable fly in the gym. And they are hovering.

Let them work in if it's not too much of a disruption to your tempo. Don't sit there staring at Instagram for three minutes in between sets. Everyone else has someplace else to be after this, too.

DON'T hover.

Let's reverse roles now. If you are the guy who wants to use the cable machine and someone else has been on it for 20 minutes, don't just hover next to it while someone else is working. Instead, wait until they are resting and then ask politely how many more sets the person has. If they are friendly (fingers crossed), then ask if you can work in. If the person using it doesn't want to let you, then find an alternative exercise. Don't "hang out" and stare at this person passive-aggressively. Recognize that this person is focused on their shit, and walk away.

Speaking of waiting until someone is resting…

DON'T talk to someone in the middle of a set.

Don't ask them to work in. Don't ask them to spot you on some other bench. Don't ask them where they got those gym shorts. Don't ask them on a date, for the time, or directions to the restroom. Don't chat. **Don't talk to someone in the middle of a lift!**

People come to the gym to work. That's why they call it "working out." (That's what I assume, anyway.) You are also there to work, not to socialize. Please do not distract me while I'm holding a dumbbell over my head.

Likewise, respect your work enough to ignore the person who doesn't get it. Concentrate on your reps. If someone talks to you mid-set, *ignore them.* You can address their concerns after you are done working. It's not personal; it's the business of lifting weights... and personal safety.

DON'T drop or slam the weights.

That loud *bang* disrupts the entire gym and throws other people off their game. Worse, you might injure yourself or someone else. This also applies to machines: don't just release your grip on that lat pull-down bar, allowing the weight stack to slam back into position. Not only is it lame and amateur, but you also risk damage to the equipment or the facility.

Treat the equipment like you own it. You would be pissed if you came in next week and the cable to your favorite machine had snapped. Why did it snap? Because someone mistreated it. *Be respectful.* Nobody thinks you're tough because you dropped a super heavy barbell on the floor. They just assume it was too much weight for you to lift correctly.

DON'T douse yourself in cologne or perfume before you go to the gym.

You're not at a nightclub. You are in close proximity to other people, and some of us will get a headache from the 25 ounces of Drakkar Noir you poured over your head. Don't do it.

Speaking of the club...

DON'T hit on strangers at the gym.

DON'T stare at that ass. DON'T whistle. And DON'T treat the gym as your sexual playground.

Please stop aggressively trying to make eye contact with me. Get the hint.

Gyms can be uncomfortable enough without having to fend off unwanted sexual pursuits. Just because a woman wears a spandex top doesn't mean she wants you to stare at her chest. *Don't be a jerk.* Focus on yourself and the work you came to do.

DON'T spread all your clothes and toiletries across the locker room so that nobody else can set their gym bag down.

And please don't consciously block other people from accessing their locker. If you are using a locker that's right next to someone else's, take your shit out of the locker and step aside so that the other person isn't waiting on your naked ass to finish spritzing Drakkar Noir on your balls. This isn't your house. We are not chillin' in your master bath. The gym is a public space, and you are not the only person using it.

Okay, I'm done.

I'm stepping off my soapbox now. Thank you for allowing me to grumble.

Also, if you have any other pet peeves or further suggestions for how humans can respect other humans at the gym, please hit me up on social media. I will commiserate with you.

Twitter: @nateclark

Instagram: @nateclarkshow

PART SIX:

THE PLANS

PUTTING IT ALL TOGETHER

This book covers a lot of information, and yet barely scratches the surface. Here it is again, boiled down to the most important advice I can provide in your quest to lose fat and gain lean muscle…

The "secret" to fat loss is math. I can't stress this enough: energy *out* must be greater than energy *in*. The small choices you make from moment to moment add up, so set small, daily goals that you can achieve regularly. Celebrate those achievements, even if they seem as simple as skipping a doughnut at breakfast. Eventually, these small wins add up to your wildest dreams. **Greatness happens NOW, not after you notice the results of your greatness. Results are merely an acknowledgment of the greatness you've already achieved.**

In order to lose fat you must maintain a caloric deficit, which means you need to burn more calories than you consume. You can achieve this by limiting the amount of food you eat, but the only way to ensure you're getting it right is to track your calories every single day. Americans routinely eat twice as many calories as they need, so we aren't talking about starving yourself. In fact, you want to avoid your body's natural "starvation response," which is why you should never eat fewer calories than indicated by your basal metabolic rate (BMR).

Have your body fat percentage tested by a professional, and use the Katch-McArdle formula to calculate your BMR. Create a daily caloric deficit based on your total daily energy expenditure (TDEE). Don't try to lose more than two pounds of fat per week. Two pounds is very aggressive, so most people will be better served by a less taxing deficit. Check changes to your weight week-over-week, and don't try to rush it. If you aren't seeing the results you want after several weeks (or months), revisit your calculations.

Don't remove any one macronutrient group from your diet. Your body depends on a mix of carbohydrate, protein, and fat to carry out its innate functions. Consuming these macros at the right times, in the correct proportions, makes it easier for you to burn fat without adding additional stress on your body or mind. Eat mindfully, with intention.

Don't rely on exercise to burn calories that you didn't need to consume in the first place. Use strength training to build muscle, or to hold on to the muscle mass you have while maintaining a caloric deficit. Train with a mix of sets for strength and sets for hypertrophy (adding muscle), and allow your muscles adequate time to rest. Focus on perfecting the form of each exercise, and remember to stretch regularly.

Use cardiovascular exercise for its intended purpose: to strengthen your heart and lungs. Add several sets of high-intensity interval training to your workout routine each week. Don't worry about how many calories you burn while doing cardio, and don't use cardio calories to "buy back" calories you've eaten. Exercise isn't an excuse to overeat.

Don't rely on supplements to reach your goals. You don't need them to lose fat. Supplements help you meet your macronutrient requirements, but they aren't a substitute for a healthy caloric deficit and regular strength training. I use supplements for convenience, not as a quick fix. Stay away from fat burners—they are dangerous—and remember that a lack of sleep impairs your ability to lose fat, so get at least seven to eight hours of sleep every night.

Remember that losing fat and gaining muscle is *math*. It's physics. The math doesn't care if you are in a bad mood or feeling blue. Emotions will fluctuate, but the math remains constant regardless of how you feel. Do the best you can *today*, with where you are *today*. Recognize that every day is a chance to succeed, and the small wins you make from day to day do add up to the body you've always dreamed of. Follow the numbers. The numbers are the only thing—THE ONLY THING—standing between you and your ultimate goals.

The following plans include 3-, 4- and 5-day splits. Use them to formulate your own strategy. If you are trying to make a radical change in your body, I suggest spending one month (four weeks) on each of these splits in succession; a total of 12 weeks. You will maximize your caloric deficit for the first four weeks while gradually ramping up to a 5-day split. The lawyers won't let me "guarantee" that you'll experience a radical change in your body by the end of those three months, but let's say it's *highly probable*.

Regardless of the approach you take, I wish you all the strength, tenacity, and patience you need. You have it in you... you just need to acknowledge it.

That's it. That's all you really need to know. **Everything else is fluff.**

3-DAY SPLIT

MONDAY: PUSH (CHEST & TRICEPS)

EXERCISE	SETS	REPS	REST	FOCUS
Bench Press (Barbell)	5	4–6	2m	Chest
Overhead Press (Barbell)	5	4–6	1m30s	Shoulders
Incline Press (Dumbbell)	4	8–10	1m	Chest
Chest Fly (Dumbbell)	4	10–12	45s	Chest
Lateral Raises	3	8–10	45s	Shoulders
Straight Bar Triceps Pushdown (Cable)	4	10–12	45s	Triceps
Push-ups	3	AMRAP*	45s	Chest

HIIT: 10 minutes, including 5 sprint intervals. Could be treadmill, rower, stair climber, etc.

TUESDAY: HIIT

HIIT: 10 minutes, including 5 sprint intervals. Bonus: add on another 10 minutes of cardio at your base pace.

CALORIC DEFICIT: Prioritize your caloric deficit. Eat as close to your BMR as possible. Minimize carb intake; if the HIIT wipes you out, increase calories with additional protein and fat.

---

* AMRAP: as many reps as possible

WEDNESDAY: LEGS & ABS

EXERCISE	SETS	REPS	REST	FOCUS
Squat (Barbell)	5	4–6	2m	Hamstrings & Glutes
Front Squat (Barbell)	4	8–10	1m	Quadriceps
Hip Thrusters (Barbell)	4	8–10	1m	Glutes
Leg Extensions (Machine)	4	10–12	45s	Quadriceps
Standing Calf Raises (Machine)	4	10–12	1m	Calves
Crunches	4	AMRAP	45s	Abdominals
Hanging Leg Raises	3–4	AMRAP	1m	Abdominals
Lower Back Extensions (Weighted)	3	15–20	45s	Lower Back

THURSDAY: STRETCH

STRETCH: Active stretching (e.g, yoga class, Pilates, etc.).

CALORIC DEFICIT: Full caloric deficit. Eat close to your BMR and minimize carbohydrate intake.

FRIDAY: PULL (BACK & BICEPS)

EXERCISE	SETS	REPS	REST	FOCUS
Deadlift (Barbell)	5	4–6	2m	Back
Lat Pull-down	5	8–10	1m	Lats
Pull-up (Assisted if needed)	4	AMRAP	1m	Lats
Dumbbell Row	4	10–12	45s	Middle Back
Preacher Curl (EZ Barbell)	4	8–10	1m	Biceps
Hammer Curls	4	8–10	1m	Biceps
Rope Curls	3	10–12	45	Biceps

HIIT: 10 minutes, including 5 sprint intervals. Could be treadmill, rower, stair climber, etc.

SATURDAY: HIIT

HIIT: 10 minutes, including 5 sprint intervals. Bonus: add on another 10 minutes of cardio at your base pace. This is an opportunity to push yourself, but don't go so far that you're tempted to screw your deficit. Your first priority today is to eat close to your BMR. If the HIIT intervals leave you starving and irritable, replace these with a long walk or something very low-impact.

CALORIC DEFICIT: Prioritize your caloric deficit. Eat close to your BMR, if possible. Minimize carb intake; if the HIIT wipes you out, increase calories with additional protein and fat.

SUNDAY: REST

STRETCH: Make time for passive stretching, such as a gentle yoga class or stretching on the floor while watching television. Don't push yourself.

CALORIC DEFICIT: Maximize caloric deficit today. Eat as close to BMR as possible (without going under) and aim for only 20% of your calories to come from carbohydrates.

WALK: Go for a long walk if possible. Again, don't push yourself to the point of getting *hangry*.

NOTES:

This 3-day split provides you with a basic strength-training routine each week while pursuing a *significant* caloric deficit. You hit each muscle group once, and you'll also spend four days each week maximizing your deficit. Aim to consume 200 or so calories below your TDEE on strength-training days. Try to consume just above your BMR on all other days.

This split groups complementary muscle groups together (e.g., "push" muscles, "pull" muscles, and legs/core.) Experiment with training opposing muscle groups when following a split like this for more than 4 weeks.

Example: **Monday:** Chest, Back, & Abs

Wednesday: Legs/Shoulders

Friday: Biceps & Triceps

Additionally, this split adds several HIIT sessions intended to boost your cardiovascular efficiency and amplify your caloric burn. But don't let those sessions tank your primary goal. If the HIIT tires you out to the point that you can't help but reach for more food, cut back on the HIIT.

4-DAY SPLIT

MONDAY: LEGS +

EXERCISE	SETS	REPS	REST	FOCUS
Squat (Barbell)	5	4–6	2m	Hamstrings & Glutes
Front Squat (Barbell)	4	8–10	1m	Quadriceps
Hip Thrust (Barbell)	4	10–12	45s	Glutes
Leg Extension (Machine)	4	10–12	45s	Quads
Preacher Curl (EZ Barbell)	5	4–6	2m	Biceps
Rope Curl	4	10–12	45s	Biceps

HIIT: 10 minutes, including 5 sprint intervals. Could be treadmill, rower, stair climber, etc.

TUESDAY: CHEST & TRICEPS

EXERCISE	SETS	REPS	REST	FOCUS
Bench Press (Barbell)	5	4–6	2m	Chest
Incline Bench Press (Barbell)	5	8–10	1m	Chest
Chest Fly (Dumbbells or Machine)	4	8–10	1m	Chest
Cable Crossover (Decline Angle)	4	10–12	45s	Chest
Overhead Triceps Extension (Dumbbell)	4	10–12	1m	Triceps
Straight Bar Triceps Pushdown (Cable)	4	10–12	1m	Triceps
Crunches	3	AMRAP*	1m	Abdominals

---

* AMRAP: as many reps as possible

WEDNESDAY: STRETCH

STRETCH: Active stretching (e.g, yoga class, Pilates, etc.).

CALORIC DEFICIT: Full caloric deficit. Eat close to your BMR and minimize carbohydrate intake.

THURSDAY: BACK & BICEPS

EXERCISE	SETS	REPS	REST	FOCUS
Deadlift (Barbell)	5	4–6	2m	Back
Pull-up (Assisted if needed)	4	AMRAP	1m	Lats
Barbell Row	4	8–10	1m	Middle Back
Lat Pull-down	4	10–12	45s	Lats
Hammer Curls	4	8–10	1m	Biceps
Push-ups	3	AMRAP	45	Chest

HIIT: 10 minutes, including 5 sprint intervals. Could be treadmill, rower, stair climber, etc.

FRIDAY: SHOULDERS +

EXERCISE	SETS	REPS	REST	FOCUS
Overhead Press (Barbell)	5	4–6	2m	Shoulders
Front Raises (Plate)	4	8–10	1m	Shoulders
Lateral Raises (Dumbbell)	4	10–12	45s	Shoulders
Dips (Weighted or assisted)	4	10–12	45s	Chest
Standing Calf Raises (Machine)	4	10–12	1m	Calves
Hanging Leg Raises	3–4	AMRAP	1m	Abdominals
Lower Back Extensions (Weighted)	2	15–20	45s	Lower Back

SATURDAY: HIIT

HIIT: 10 minutes, including 5 sprint intervals. Bonus: add on another 10 minutes of cardio at your base pace. Push yourself hard on these intervals. You'll be resting until Monday.

CALORIC DEFICIT: Prioritize your caloric deficit today. Minimize carb intake; if the HIIT wipes you out, increase calories with additional protein and fat.

SUNDAY: REST

STRETCH: Make time for passive stretching, such as a gentle yoga class or stretching on the floor while watching television. DO NOT push yourself; you aren't attempting to increase your flexibility.

CALORIC DEFICIT: Maximize caloric deficit today. Eat as close to BMR as possible (without going under) and aim for only 20% of your calories to come from carbohydrates.

WALK: Go for a long walk if possible, but don't push yourself.

NOTES:

This 4-day split hits a sweet spot between maximizing your caloric deficit and a hypertrophic approach to weight training. Four days of training provides ample opportunity to hit every muscle group at least once. You'll also spend three days—nearly half the week—maximizing your caloric deficit. This split is still intended for fat loss, so that should be your primary objective.

Additionally, this split adds a few additional sets for unrelated muscle groups on Monday and Friday. I call these "+" sets. You can swap those exercises to target other muscle groups that might be trouble spots for you. Just try to provide ample rest time between sessions where you train the same muscles, even if you only do one or two sets for that muscle group.

As mentioned before, the focus muscles listed are where I suggest you put the mind-muscle connection. Use these reps to build the muscles listed, even though you're certain to engage other muscles as well.

5-DAY SPLIT

MONDAY: LEGS & BICEPS

EXERCISE	SETS	REPS	REST	FOCUS
Squat (Barbell)	5	4–6	2m	Hamstrings & Glutes
Leg Press (Machine)	4	8–10	1m	Hamstrings & Glutes
Hip Thrust (Barbell)	4	10–12	1m	Glutes
Leg Curl (Machine)	4	10–12	45s	Hamstrings
Biceps Curl (Barbell)	5	4–6	2m	Biceps
Incline Biceps Curl (Dumbbell)	4	10–12	1m	Biceps
Reverse Grip Biceps Curl (Cable or Dumbbell)	3	10–12	45s	Biceps

TUESDAY: CHEST & TRICEPS

EXERCISE	SETS	REPS	REST	FOCUS
Bench Press (Barbell)	5	4–6	2m	Chest
Incline Bench Press (Dumbbell)	4	8–10	1m	Chest
Chest Fly (Dumbbells or Machine)	4	8–10	1m	Chest
Cable Crossover	4	10–12	45s	Chest
Overhead Triceps Extension (Dumbbell)	4	10–12	1m	Triceps
Straight Bar Triceps Pushdown (Cable)	4	10–12	1m	Triceps

HIIT: 10 minutes, including at least 5 sprint intervals. Could be treadmill, rower, stair-climber, etc., depending on how tired your legs are from yesterday.

BONUS: Additional 10 minutes of cardio at your "base pace" after the sprint intervals.

WEDNESDAY: BACK & CORE

EXERCISE	SETS	REPS	REST	FOCUS
Bent-Over Row (Barbell)	4	4–6	2m	Middle Back
Pull-ups (Weighted or assisted)	5	AMRAP*	1m	Lats
Lat Pull-down - Wide Grip (Cable)	4	10–12	1m	Lats
Single Arm Row (Dumbbell)	4	10–12	45s	Lats
Rope Crunches	4	10–12	1m	Abdominals
Lower Back Extensions (Weighted)	2	15–20	45s	Lower Back

HIIT: 10 minutes, including at least 5 sprint intervals. Try something different from the previous day, if possible.

THURSDAY: REST

STRETCH: Make time for passive stretching, such as a gentle yoga class or stretching on the floor while watching television. Don't push yourself; you aren't attempting to increase your flexibility.

WALK: Keep moving, but don't think of it as "cardio." Go for a long walk if possible.

CALORIC DEFICIT: Prioritize your caloric deficit. Consume at or just above your BMR if possible. You aren't training, so you'll need fewer carbohydrates and fewer calories overall.

FRIDAY: LEGS 2 & ABS

EXERCISE	SETS	REPS	REST	FOCUS
Deadlift (Barbell)	5	4–6	2m	Hamstrings
Front Squats (Barbell)	4	8–10	2m	Quadriceps
Leg Extension (Machine)	4	8–10	1m	Quadriceps
Bulgarian Split Squat (Dumbbell)	4	10–12	1m	Quadriceps
Standing Calf Raises (Machine)	4	10–12	1m	Calves
Hanging Leg Raises	3–4	AMRAP	45s	Abdominals
Crunches	3–4	AMRAP	45s	Abdominals

---

* AMRAP: as many reps as possible

SATURDAY: SHOULDERS & ARMS

EXERCISE	SETS	REPS	REST	FOCUS
Standing Military Press (Barbell)	5	4–6	2m	Shoulders
Seated Shoulder Press (Dumbbell)	4	8–10	1m	Shoulders
Lateral Raise (Dumbbell)	4	10–12	1m	Shoulders
Rear Delt Fly (Machine or Dumbbells)	4	10–12	1m	Rear Shoulders
Preacher Curl (EZ Barbell)	3–4	10–12	1m	Biceps
V-Bar Triceps Extension (Cable)	3–4	10–12	45s	Abdominals

HIIT: 10 to 20 minutes, including at least 5 sprint intervals. Get your heart rate up, for real!

SUNDAY: REST

STRETCH: Consider an active stretching class today (e.g., yoga, Pilates, etc.), but don't push yourself too hard. If you need to rest completely, honor that.

CALORIC DEFICIT: Like all rest days, you aren't training so you need fewer carbohydrates and fewer calories overall. Don't think of this rest day as a "cheat day." You're resting your muscles, but you aren't resting your goals!

NOTES:

This 5-day split prioritizes legs and biceps while also hitting every other major muscle group throughout the week. Use it as a template and substitute other muscle groups if training legs isn't your focus.

This split isn't as "aggressive" as many other 5-day splits, but it's allowed me to grow a bit while also maintaining a deficit. Two days of a larger caloric deficit each week probably isn't enough for dramatic fat loss, but this split favors muscle maintenance over losing fat. If you're close to your ideal body fat percentage, or if you're tired after a more intense cutting phase, this split is a terrific foundation for specialized muscle training without going into a full-on bulking phase.

Maximize your deficit on rest days, and maintain a smaller caloric deficit (200 to 300 calories) on training days.

PREFERRED EXERCISES

Here's a list of my preferred exercises, grouped by body part. For the compound exercises I've indicated the muscles I typically focus on. That doesn't mean you can't do something else, it's just where I set my intention (i.e., the mind-muscle connection). Note that almost all back exercises are technically compound exercises, because it's difficult to isolate the muscles in the back. Conversely, dedicated arm exercises are isolation exercises.

I've indicated abdominal exercises as a simple list, in lieu of separating them by target area. It's not important to spend too much time specializing at this stage of the game, especially if your primary focus is to lose fat. Also, standard planks are garbage, so don't let some lazy trainer force you to hold a plank for five minutes.

I've indicated my preferred method—barbell, dumbbell, etc.—for the exercises that call for that. Yes, I know there are many other variations, many other exercises, and everyone has an opinion about what they like best. But these are the exercises I prefer, and I'm confident they provide a solid foundation for any training program. Don't @ me.

LEGS

EXERCISE	TYPE	FOCUS	SECONDARY
Squat, a.k.a. "Back Squat" or Standard Squat (Barbell)	Compound	Hamstrings or Glutes	Quadriceps, Calves, Core
Front Squat (Barbell)	Compound	Quadriceps	Hamstrings, Glutes, Calves, Lower Back
Bulgarian Split Squat (Dumbbell)	Compound	Quadriceps	Glutes
Hip Thrusters (Barbell)	Isolation	Glutes	Hamstrings

Leg Extensions (Machine)	Isolation	Quadriceps	
Leg Curl, a.k.a Hamstring Curl (Machine)	Isolation	Hamstrings	
Standing Calf Raises (Machine)	Isolation	Calves	

CHEST

EXERCISE	TYPE	FOCUS	SECONDARY
Bench Press (Barbell)	Compound	Pectorals	Triceps, Shoulders
Dips	Compound	Pectorals	Triceps, Shoulders
Incline Press (Barbell)	Compound	Pectorals (Upper)	Triceps, Shoulders
Incline Press (Dumbbell)	Compound	Pectorals (Upper)	Triceps, Shoulders
Decline Press (Barbell)	Compound	Pectorals (Lower)	Triceps, Shoulders
Push-up	Compound	Pectorals	Triceps, Shoulders
Chest Fly (Dumbbell)	Isolation	Pectorals (Mid Inner)	
Cable Crossover	Isolation	Pectorals (Mid Inner)	
Incline Chest Fly (Dumbbell)	Isolation	Pectorals (Upper Inner)	

BACK

EXERCISE	TYPE	FOCUS	SECONDARY
Standard Deadlift (Barbell)	Compound	Back (Lower and Mid) or Glutes	Hamstrings, Quads, Shoulders, Core
Pull-ups (Palms Out)	Compound	Back (Most Muscles)	Biceps
Bent-Over Barbell Row	Compound	Back (Most Muscles)	Biceps

Lat Pull-down	Isolation	Lats	
Single-Arm Dumbbell Row	Compound	Lats (Lower)	Biceps
Lat Pull-over	Isolation	Lats	
Lower Back Extension	Isolation	Lower Back	

ARMS

EXERCISE	FOCUS
Biceps Curl (Barbell)	Biceps
Preacher Curl (EZ Curl Bar)	Biceps
Hammer Curl (Dumbbell)	Biceps
Wide-grip Barbell Curl (Barbell)	Biceps
Reverse Cable Curl (Cable)	Biceps
Rope Curl (Cable)	Biceps
Triceps Extension (Barbell)	Triceps
Triceps Extension (Dumbbell)	Triceps
Triceps Pushdown (Straight Bar on Cable)	Triceps
Triceps Rope Pushdown	Triceps
Reverse Triceps Extension (Cable)	Triceps
Reverse Wrist Curl (Barbell)	Forearms

SHOULDERS

EXERCISE	TYPE	FOCUS	SECONDARY
Overhead Press (Barbell)	Compound	Deltoids (Shoulders)	Pecs, Trapezius, Triceps
Lateral Raise (Dumbbell)	Isolation	Deltoids (Shoulders)	
Front Raise (Plate)	Isolation	Deltoids (Shoulders)	
Rear Delt Fly (Dumbbells)	Isolation	Rear Deltoids	
External Shoulder Rotation (Cable)	Isolation	External Rotators	
Handstand Push-ups	Compound	Deltoids (Shoulders)	Pecs, Trapezius, Triceps, Core

ABDOMINALS / CORE

Standard Crunch

Rope Crunch

Hanging Leg Raise

RKC Plank

Side Plank

V-up

Lying Leg Raise

Bicycle Crunch

Russian Twist

Bird Dog

Hollow Hold

GROCERY SHOPPING LIST

Below is a list of foods I eat on the regular. I've listed the carbs (carbohydrate dense) foods in order of ascending glycemic load, and I've also indicated the serving size and glycemic index for each of these foods. Please note: this data is based on various studies[100] and is point-in-time specific for various individuals. There is a standard error of the mean for most of the GI numbers ranging from ±1 to ±10. That is to say, *these numbers are merely a guideline to help you plan your carbohydrate intake according to your activity levels and needs.* You should also take into account the amount of sugar, fiber, and the volume of these servings when planning what to eat. Use your calories tracker of choice for that. If you'd like more detailed information about the glucose tolerance of many foods, check out the *International Tables of Glycemic Index and Glycemic Load Values: 2008.*

Yes, I've included rice pasta and popcorn on this list and yes, I know they are technically processed grains. *I'm doing the best I can over here!*

CARBS

FOOD	SERVING	GI	GL	CATEGORY
Carrots (raw)	80 g	35	2	VEGETABLE
Lentils (red)	150 g	21	4	LEGUME
Orange (raw)	120 g	40	4	FRUIT
Watermelon	120 g	72	4	FRUIT
Green Peas	80 g	51	4	VEGETABLE
Apple	120 g	24	6	FRUIT
Kidney Beans	150 g	25	6	LEGUME
Pineapple (raw)	120 g	66	6	FRUIT

Popcorn	20 g	55	6	SNACK
Apricots (dried)	60 g	30	7	FRUIT
Mango (raw)	120 g	51	8	FRUIT
Banana	120 g	47	11	FRUIT
Chickpeas (boiled)	150 g	36	11	LEGUME
Steel Cut Oats (cooked)	250 g	57	14	CEREALS
Corn (on the cob, boiled)	150 g	48	14	GRAIN
Honey (clover)	25 g	69	15	SUGARS
Barley (boiled)	150 g	35	15	GRAIN
Dates (raw)	60 g	36	16	FRUIT
Russet Potato (unpeeled, baked)	120 g	77	19	VEGETABLE
White Rice (long grain, pre-cooked)	150 g	52	19	GRAIN
Brown Rice	150 g	48	20	GRAIN
Rice Pasta (gluten-free)	180 g	51	24	HIGH-CARB FOOD
Raisins	120 g	64	28	FRUIT
Sweet Potato (peeled, baked)	150 g	94	42	VEGETABLE
Taro (peeled, boiled)	150 g	53	75	VEGETABLE

VEGETABLES

The following vegetables—mostly leafy green and cruciferous—are typically a safe choice at any time of the day. As long as you don't cover them in oil or butter. These are my personal favorites.

Arugula	Cabbage
Asparagus	Cauliflower
Bell Peppers	Kale
Broccoli	Spinach
Brussels Sprouts	Tomato*
Butter Lettuce	Turnips

---

* Technically a fruit. I know, I know.

PROTEINS

Casein Protein Powder	Salmon
Chicken Breast (skinless)	Shark
Eggs	Shrimp
Halibut	Tuna**
Lean Ground Turkey (90%)	Turkey Breast
Liquid Egg Whites	Whey Protein Powder

FATS

The following foods add fat to your diet. Some of them are high-fat foods and others are fats you can add to your meals. A little fat goes a long way, so eat these in moderation based on your macronutrient goals, and balance them against the fat content in other foods.

Almonds (dry roasted, salted)	Ground Walnuts
Avocado	Natural Nut Butters (just nuts! no added sugar or oil)
Avocado Oil	Olive Oil
Chia Seeds	Olives
Coconut	Omega-3 Supplement (various)
Ground Flaxseed	Whole Eggs

** Be mindful of mercury intake.

ACKNOWLEDGMENTS

I wouldn't have been able to finish this book without the support of my husband, Allen. Not only because he let me hole up in the office while he changed diapers, walked the dogs, made dinner (after he got home from buying the groceries), and did everything else when I opted to write. I'm also grateful because he never shames me when he finds an empty Häagen-Dazs container in the trash or notices that all three jars of Kirkland brand peanut butter have disappeared in less than a week. He's the most supportive, loving, patient partner a person could want. This book wouldn't exist without him. (I love you, mister.)

I'd also like to thank my dad for modeling a lifelong dedication to physical fitness. He's been going to the gym at least three or four days a week for 50-some years… since before gyms had running water or air conditioning, I think. (I'm pretty sure he started training by lifting rocks in a cave.) He's always made fitness a priority, and he's showed me the value of it since I was a kid. Even though I didn't always pay attention.

Thanks to Jessica Hatch for editorial guidance and positive energy, and Diane Szulecki for further editorial assistance. And thanks to colleagues and collaborators at Snazzy Co. for continued support.

I also want to give a big shout-out to all the trainers, coaches, dietitians, fitness gurus, and hacks I've met along the way. Some of your advice is in this book, and some of it really screwed me up! Regardless, I'm grateful to you all for the countless opportunities I've had to try (and fail) to get in shape. You've made me wiser, stronger, and more adept at sniffing out bullshit.

Finally, a sincere thanks to the friends and strangers who kept asking me, "Hey, how did you lose the fat? Send me your plan!" You have all been so incredibly kind and you've truly made me feel like a million bucks. Anyway, you asked, so here it is. I hope it has all the answers you are looking for.

And if it doesn't… maybe try Barry's?

NOTES

1 Pasco, Julie A., Kara L. Holloway, Amelia G. Dobbins, et al. "Body Mass Index and Measures of Body Fat for Defining Obesity and Underweight: A Cross-Sectional, Population-Based Study." BMC Obesity. 1. June 2014. https://doi.org/10.1186/2052-9538-1-9.

2 McDowell, Margaret A., Cheryl D. Fryar, Cynthia L. Ogden, and Katherine M. Flegal. "Anthropometric Reference Data for Children and Adults: United States, 2003-2006." National Health Statistics Reports. 10. October 2008. https://doi.org/10.1037/e623932009-001.

3 Maffetone, Philip B., and Paul B. Laursen. "The Prevalence of Overfat Adults and Children in the US." Frontiers in Public Health. 5. November 2017. https://doi.org/10.3389/fpubh.2017.00290.

4 Maffetone, Philip B., Ivan Rivera-Dominguez, and Paul B. Laursen. 2017. "Overfat and Underfat: New Terms and Definitions Long Overdue." Frontiers in Public Health. 4 (January). https://doi.org/10.3389/fpubh.2016.00279.

5 Moore, Justin Xavier, Ninad Chaudhary, and Tomi Akinyemiju. "Metabolic Syndrome Prevalence by Race/Ethnicity and Sex in the United States, National Health and Nutrition Examination Survey, 1988–2012." Preventing Chronic Disease. 14. March 2017. https://doi.org/10.5888/pcd14.160287.

6 Pi-sunyer, Xavier, Robert H. Eckel, Paul Poirier, Thomas D. Giles, George A. Bray, Yuling Hong, Judith S. Stern, et al. 2005. On Obesity and Heart Disease From the Obesity Committee of the Council.

7 Benjamin, Emelia J., Paul Muntner, Alvaro Alonso, et al. "Heart Disease and Stroke Statistics—2019 Update: A Report From the American Heart Association." Circulation. 139(10). March 2019. www.ahajournals.org/doi/full/10.1161/CIR.0000000000000659.

8 Rowley, William R., Clement Bezold, Yasemin Arikan, Erin Byrne, and Shannon Krohe. "Diabetes 2030: Insights from Yesterday, Today, and Future Trends." Population Health Management. 20(1): 6–12. February 2017. https://doi.org/10.1089/pop.2015.0181.

9 Food and Agriculture Organization of the United Nations (FAOUN). World Food and Agriculture: Statistical Pocketbook 2018., 2018. [227].

10 "Average Number of Calories Americans Eat Has Increased Dramatically - Business Insider." https://www.businessinsider.com/daily-calories-americans-eat-increase-2016-07.

11 FAOUN (n9) [46]

12 "SNICKERS® ORIGINAL SINGLE." n.d. Accessed November 25, 2019. https://marschocolate.com/snickers/snickers-original-single.

13 "DORITOS® Nacho Cheese Flavored Tortilla Chips | Doritos." n.d. Accessed November 25, 2019. http://www.doritos.com/products/doritos-nacho-cheese-flavored-tortilla-chips.

14 "Starbucks®." n.d. Accessed November 25, 2019. https://www.starbucks.com/menu/product/408/hot?parent=%2Fdrinks%2Fhot-coffees%2Fmochas.

15 "Teasing Kids About Their Weight May Make Them Gain More." n.d. NPR.org. Accessed November 25, 2019. https://www.npr.org/sections/health-shots/2019/05/30/728111494/teasing-kids-about-their-weight-may-make-them-gain-more.

16 Einstein, Albert. Relativity: The Special and the General Theory. Trans. Robert W. Lawson. New York: Henry Holt and Company, 1921.

17 Peterson, Hayley. "A Teacher Who Lost 56 Pounds Eating Only McDonald's Is Starring in a Documentary to Show Kids about 'Healthy' Eating." Business Insider. October 13, 2015. Accessed October 27, 2019. https://www.businessinsider.com/how-to-lose-weight-eating-only-mcdonalds-2015-10.

18 Mettler, Fred A., Walter Huda, Terry T. Yoshizumi, and Mahadevappa Mahesh. "Effective Doses in Radiology and Diagnostic Nuclear Medicine: A Catalog." Radiology. 248(1): 254–63. July 1, 2008. https://doi.org/10.1148/radiol.2481071451.

19 "Bone Densitometry (DEXA , DXA)." Radiology Society of North America, Inc. Reviewed August 10, 2018. Accessed October 27, 2019. www.radiologyinfo.org/en/info.cfm?pg=dexa.

20 "The Water in You: Water and the Human Body." U.S. Department of the Interior. Accessed October 27, 2019. www.usgs.gov/special-topic/water-science-school/science/water-you-water-and-human-body?qt-science_center_objects=0#qt-science_center_objects.

21 Kyle, Ursula G., Ingvar Bosaeus, Antonio D. De Lorenzo, Paul Deurenberg, Marinos Elia, José Manuel Gómez, Berit Lilienthal Heitmann, et al. 2004. "Bioelectrical Impedance Analysis—Part I: Review of Principles and Methods." Clinical Nutrition 23 (5): 1226–43. https://doi.org/10.1016/j.clnu.2004.06.004.

22 "Bioelectrical Impedance Analysis in Body Composition Measurement." National Institutes of Health Technology Assessment Conference Statement. December 12-14, 1994. Accessed October 27, 2019. https://consensus.nih.gov/1994/1994BioelectricImpedanceBodyta015html.htm.

23 Ling, Carolina H. Y., Anton J. M. de Craen, Pieternella E. Slagboom, Dave A. Gunn, Marcel P. M. Stokkel, Rudi G. J. Westendorp, and Andrea B. Maier. 2011. "Accuracy of Direct Segmental Multi-Frequency Bioimpedance Analysis in the Assessment of Total Body and Segmental Body Composition in Middle-Aged Adult Population." Clinical Nutrition 30 (5): 610–15. https://doi.org/10.1016/j.clnu.2011.04.001.

24 Bod Pod is a registered trademark of COSMED USA, INC. The author, Fitnrd, and Snazzy Co, LLC are not affiliated with this brand in any way.

25 "COSMED–BOD POD–Air Displacement Plethysmograph." n.d. Accessed December 2, 2019. https://www.cosmed.com/en/products/body-composition/bod-pod.

26 Venuto, Tom. "Starvation Mode Revisited: Is This the Cause of Slow Fat Loss, Frustrating Plateaus And Weight Re-Gain?" Burn the Fat Blog. Accessed October 27, 2019. www.burnthefatblog.com/archives/2012/12/starvation-mode-revisited.php.

27 Rosenbaum, Michael, and Rudolph L. Leibel. "Adaptive Thermogenesis in Humans." International Journal of Obesity. 34(1):S47–S55. October 2010. https://doi.org/10.1038/ijo.2010.184.

28   Rosenbaum, Michael, Jules Hirsch, Dympna A. Gallagher, and Rudolph L. Leibel. 2008. "Long-Term Persistence of Adaptive Thermogenesis in Subjects Who Have Maintained a Reduced Body Weight." The American Journal of Clinical Nutrition 88 (4): 906–12. https://doi.org/10.1093/ajcn/88.4.906.

29   Fothergill, Erin, Juen Guo, Lilian Howard, Jennifer C. Kerns, Nicolas D. Knuth, Robert Brychta, Kong Y. Chen, et al. 2016. "Persistent Metabolic Adaptation 6 Years after 'The Biggest Loser' Competition." Obesity 24 (8): 1612–19. https://doi.org/10.1002/oby.21538.

30   Hall, Kevin D. "What Is the Required Energy Deficit per Unit Weight Loss?" International Journal of Obesity. 32(3): 573–76. March 2008. https://doi.org/10.1038/sj.ijo.0803720.

31   "Adenosine Triphosphate | Definition, Structure, Function, & Facts." n.d. Encyclopedia Britannica. Accessed December 6, 2019. https://www.britannica.com/science/adenosine-triphosphate.

32   "Food Energy and ATP | Biology for Majors II." n.d. Accessed December 6, 2019. https://courses.lumenlearning.com/wm-biology2/chapter/food-energy-and-atp/.

33   "Insulin Resistance & Prediabetes | NIDDK." n.d. National Institute of Diabetes and Digestive and Kidney Diseases. Accessed December 3, 2019. https://www.niddk.nih.gov/health-information/diabetes/overview/what-is-diabetes/prediabetes-insulin-resistance.

34   "Diet and Insulin Resistance: Foods to Eat and Diet Tips." n.d. Medical News Today. Accessed December 3, 2019. https://www.medicalnewstoday.com/articles/316569.php.

35   Paoli, Antonio, Laura Mancin, Antonino Bianco, Ewan Thomas, João Felipe Mota, and Fabio Piccini. "Ketogenic Diet and Microbiota: Friends or Enemies?" Genes 10, no. 7 (July 15, 2019). https://doi.org/10.3390/genes10070534.

36   Agans, Richard, Alex Gordon, Denise Lynette Kramer, Sergio Perez-Burillo, José A. Rufián-Henares, and Oleg Paliy. "Dietary Fatty Acids Sustain the Growth of the Human Gut Microbiota." Edited by Edward G. Dudley. Applied and Environmental Microbiology 84, no. 21 (September 21, 2018): e01525-18, /aem/84/21/e01525-18.atom. https://doi.org/10.1128/AEM.01525-18.

37   Hernández-Alonso, Pablo, Jordi Salas-Salvadó, Miguel Ruiz-Canela, Dolores Corella, Ramón Estruch, Montserrat Fitó, Fernando Arós, et al. 2016. "High Dietary Protein Intake Is Associated with an Increased Body Weight and Total Death Risk." Clinical Nutrition 35 (2): 496–506. https://doi.org/10.1016/j.clnu.2015.03.016.

38   Pan, An, Qi Sun, Adam M. Bernstein, Matthias B. Schulze, JoAnn E. Manson, Meir J. Stampfer, Walter C. Willett, and Frank B. Hu. 2012. "Red Meat Consumption and Mortality: Results From 2 Prospective Cohort Studies." Archives of Internal Medicine 172 (7): 555–63. https://doi.org/10.1001/archinternmed.2011.2287.

39   Cuenca-Sánchez, Marta, Diana Navas-Carrillo, and Esteban Orenes-Piñero. 2015. "Controversies Surrounding High-Protein Diet Intake: Satiating Effect and Kidney and Bone Health." Advances in Nutrition 6 (3): 260–66. https://doi.org/10.3945/an.114.007716.

40   Fink, Howard A., Joseph W. Akornor, Pranav S. Garimella, Rod MacDonald, Andrea Cutting, Indulis R. Rutks, Manoj Monga, and Timothy J. Wilt. 2009. "Diet, Fluid, or Supplements for Secondary Prevention of Nephrolithiasis: A Systematic Review and Meta-Analysis of Randomized Trials." European Urology 56 (1): 72–80. https://doi.org/10.1016/j.eururo.2009.03.031.

41   Manore, Melinda M. 2005. "Exercise and the Institute of Medicine Recommendations for Nutrition." Current Sports Medicine Reports 4 (4): 193–98. https://doi.org/10.1097/01.csmr.0000306206.72186.00.

42   "A Closer Look Inside Healthy Eating Patterns–2015-2020 Dietary Guidelines–Health. Gov." n.d. Accessed December 4, 2019. https://health.gov/dietaryguidelines/2015/guidelines/chapter-1/a-closer-look-inside-healthy-eating-patterns/#table-1-1.

43 "Physical Activity Calorie Counter." The American Council on Exercise. Accessed October 28, 2019. www.acefitness.org/education-and-resources/lifestyle/tools-calculators/physical-activity-calorie-counter.

44 Breslau, Ellen. "9 Hidden Sources Of Sugar In Your Diet." HuffPost. Updated December 6, 2017. Accessed October 28, 2019. www.huffpost.com/entry/hidden-sugar-in-food-_n_7020234.

45 Whole30 (https://whole30.com) is a registered trademark of Thirty & Co, LLC. The author, Fitnrd, and Snazzy Co, LLC are not affiliated with this brand in any way.

46 Gunn, Tina. "'Bread Head' – Preventing Alzheimer's at Checkout." A Place for Mom. February 16, 2015. www.alzheimers.net/2-16-15-bread-head-prevent-alzheimers/.

47 Schilling, Melissa A. "Unraveling Alzheimer's: Making Sense of the Relationship between Diabetes and Alzheimer's Disease." Journal of Alzheimer's Disease. 51(4): 961–77. 2016. https://doi.org/10.3233/JAD-150980.

48 Belluck, Pam. 2019. "Why Didn't She Get Alzheimer's? The Answer Could Hold a Key to Fighting the Disease." The New York Times, November 4, 2019, sec. Health. https://www.nytimes.com/2019/11/04/health/alzheimers-treatment-genetics.html.

49 Atkinson, Fiona S., Kaye Foster-Powell, and Jennie C. Brand-Miller. "International Tables of Glycemic Index and Glycemic Load Values: 2008." Diabetes Care. 31(12): 2281–83. December 2008. [Table A1, A2] https://doi.org/10.2337/dc08-1239.

50 "Got Lactase?" Understanding Evolution. April 2007. Accessed October 28, 2019. https://evolution.berkeley.edu/evolibrary/news/070401_lactose.

51 Tishkoff, Sarah A., Floyd A. Reed, Alessia Ranciaro, et al. "Convergent Adaptation of Human Lactase Persistence in Africa and Europe." Nature Genetics. 39: 31–40. January 2007. https://doi.org/10.1038/ng1946.

52 Strawbridge, Holly. "Artificial Sweeteners: Sugar-Free, but at What Cost?" Harvard Health Publishing. Updated January 8, 2018. www.health.harvard.edu/blog/artificial-sweeteners-sugar-free-but-at-what-cost-201207165030.

53 Nordqvist, Joseph. "Artificial Sweeteners Affect Metabolism and Insulin Levels." Medical News Today. May 30, 2013. Accessed October 28, 2019. www.medicalnewstoday.com/articles/261179.php.

54 Paddock, Catharine. "Artificial Sweeteners Could Make You Gain Weight, Study." Medical News Today. February 11, 2008. Accessed October 28, 2019. www.medicalnewstoday.com/articles/96849.php.

55 Ferris, Robert. "Diet Soda May Not Be Any Better for You." Business Insider. July 15, 2013. Accessed October 28, 2019. www.businessinsider.com/diet-soda-may-not-be-any-better-for-you-2013-7.

56 This book is not advice meant for teenagers; if you're reading this book hoping to lose weight under the age of 18, talk to your parents, your therapist, or a guidance counselor.

57 Avena, Nicole M., Pedro Rada, and Bartley G. Hoebel. "Evidence for Sugar Addiction: Behavioral and Neurochemical Effects of Intermittent, Excessive Sugar Intake." Neuroscience and Biobehavioral Reviews. 32(1): 20–39. 2008. https://doi.org/10.1016/j.neubiorev.2007.04.019.

58 Hebebrand, Johannes, Özgür Albayrak, Roger Adan, et al. "'Eating Addiction', Rather than 'Food Addiction', Better Captures Addictive-like Eating Behavior." Neuroscience & Biobehavioral Reviews. 47: 295-306. November 2014. Accessed October 29, 2019. https://doi.org/10.1016/j.neubiorev.2014.08.016.

59 "Incentives and Disincentives for Reducing Sugar in Manufactured Foods (2017)." World Health Organization Regional Office for Europe. www.euro.who.int/en/health-topics/disease-prevention/nutrition/publications/2017/incentives-and-disincentives-for-reducing-sugar-in-manufactured-foods-2017.

60   Magee, Elaine. "8 Ways to Burn Calories and Fight Fat." WebMD. Accessed October 30, 2019. www.webmd.com/diet/obesity/features/8-ways-to-burn-calories-and-fight-fat.

61   Ginis, Kathleen A. Martin, Rebecca L. Bassett-Gunter, and Catherine Conlin. "Body Image and Exercise." The Oxford Handbook of Exercise Psychology. May 2012. https://doi.org/10.1093/oxfor dhb/9780195394313.013.0004.

62   Seguin, Rebecca, Galen Eldridge, Wesley Lynch, and Lynn Paul. "Strength Training Improves Body Image and Physical Activity Behaviors Among Midlife and Older Rural Women." Journal of Extension. 51(4): AFEA2. August 2013. Accessed October 30, 2019. https://joe.org/joe/2013august/a2.php.

63   Strickland, Justin C., and Mark A. Smith. "The Anxiolytic Effects of Resistance Exercise." Frontiers in Psychology. 5:753. July 10, 2014. https://doi.org/10.3389/fpsyg.2014.00753.

64   Wasmer Andrews, Linda. "How Strength Training Helps Keep Anxiety at Bay." Psychology Today. March 29, 2017. Accessed October 30, 2019. www.psychologytoday.com/blog/minding-the-body/201703/ how-strength-training-helps-keep-anxiety-bay.

65   Fetters, K. Aleisha. "11 Benefits of Strength Training That Have Nothing to Do with Muscle Size." U.S. News and World Report. March 23, 2018. Accessed October 30, 2019. https://health.usnews. com/wellness/fitness/articles/ 2018-03-23/11-benefits-of-strength-training-that-have-nothing-to-do-with-muscle-size.

66   National Institute on Drug Abuse. n.d. "What Is the History of Anabolic Steroid Use?" Accessed December 6, 2019. https://www.drugabuse.gov/publications/research-reports/ steroids-other-appearance-performance-enhancing-drugs-apeds/what-history-anabolic-steroid-use.

67   Brad J. Schoenfeld, Dan Ogborn, and James W. Krieger (2017). The dose–response relationship between resistance training volume and muscle hypertrophy: are there really still any doubts?, Journal of Sports Sciences, 35:20, 1985-1987, DOI: 10.1080/02640414.2016.1243800

68   Shaner, Aaron A., Jakob L. Vingren, Disa L. Hatfield, Ronald G. Budnar Jr., Anthony A. Duplanty, and David W. Hill. 2014. "The Acute Hormonal Response to Free Weight and Machine Weight Resistance Exercise." The Journal of Strength & Conditioning Research 28 (4): 1032–1039..

69   Narici, M. V., G. S. Roi, L. Landoni, A. E. Minetti, and P. Cerretelli. "Changes in Force, Cross-Sectional Area and Neural Activation during Strength Training and Detraining of the Human Quadriceps." European Journal of Applied Physiology and Occupational Physiology. 59(4): 310–19. November 1989. https://doi.org/10.1007/ BF02388334.

70   Pearson, A.M. "Muscle Growth and Exercise" *Critical Reviews in Food Science and Nutrition.* 29(3): 167-196. 1990. Accessed November 1, 2019. www.tandfonline.com/doi/abs/10.1080/10408399009527522.

71   Schoenfeld, Brad J., Bret Contreras, James Krieger, et al. "Resistance Training Volume Enhances Muscle Hypertrophy but Not Strength in Trained Men." *Medicine & Science in Sports and Exercise.* 51(1): 94–103. January 2019. https://doi.org/10.1249/MSS.0000000000001764.

72   Grimsby, Ola, and Jim Rivard. *Science, Theory and Clinical Application in Orthopaedic Manual Physical Therapy: Applied Science and Theory.* The Academy of Graduate Physical Therapy, 2009. Lulu.com.

73   "Low Back Pain Fact Sheet." National Institute of Neurological Disorders and Stroke. Updated August 13, 2019. Accessed November 1, 2019. www.ninds.nih.gov/Disorders/Patient-Caregiver-Education/ Fact-Sheets/Low-Back-Pain-Fact-Sheet.

74   Daneshmandi, Hadi, Alireza Choobineh, Haleh Ghaem, and Mehran Karimi. "Adverse Effects of Prolonged Sitting Behavior on the General Health of Office Workers." Journal of Lifestyle Medicine. 7(2): 69–75. July 2017. https://doi.org/10.15280/jlm.2017.7.2.69.

75 Raphael, Rina. "Stretching Studios Are the Next Big Boutique Fitness Trend." Fast Company, November 27, 2018. https://www.fastcompany.com/90269526/stretching-studios-are-the-next-big-boutique-fitness-trend.

76 DiMaggio, Robert. "Overtrain If You Don't Want To Gain!" Bodybuilding.com. Updated January 18, 2019. www.bodybuilding.com/fun/dimaggio12.htm.

77 Graves, J. E., M. L. Pollock, S. H. Leggett, R. W. Braith, D. M. Carpenter, and L. E. Bishop. "Effect of Reduced Training Frequency on Muscular Strength." International Journal of Sports Medicine 9, no. 5 (October 1988): 316–19.

78 DeRenne, Coop, Ronald K. Hetzler, Barton P. Buxton, and Kwok W. Ho. "Effects of Training Frequency on Strength Maintenance in Pubescent Baseball Players." The Journal of Strength & Conditioning Research 10, no. 1 (February 1996): 8–14.

79 Schoenfeld, Brad J., Bret Contreras, James Krieger, Jozo Grgic, Kenneth Delcastillo, Ramon Belliard, and Andrew Alto. "Resistance Training Volume Enhances Muscle Hypertrophy but Not Strength in Trained Men." Medicine and Science in Sports and Exercise 51, no. 1 (2019): 94–103.

80 "10 Great Reasons to Love Aerobic Exercise." n.d. Mayo Clinic. Accessed December 7, 2019. https://www.mayoclinic.org/healthy-lifestyle/fitness/in-depth/aerobic-exercise/art-20045541.

81 Bonner, Herman. "5 Reasons to Boost Your VO2max." Firstbeat. 2019. Accessed November 2, 2019. www.firstbeat.com/en/blog/5-reasons-boost-vo2max/.

82 Petter, Olivia. "Why Cardio Is Better for Your Metabolism than Strength Training." The Independent. August 25, 2018. www.independent.co.uk/life-style/health-and-families/cardio-strength-training-metabolism-effect-study-university-of-copenhagan-a8507641.html.

83 "JCI Insight–Divergent Effects of Resistance and Endurance Exercise on Plasma Bile Acids, FGF19, and FGF21 in Humans." n.d. Accessed November 2, 2019. https://insight.jci.org/articles/view/122737.

84 "Starbucks®." n.d. Accessed December 8, 2019. https://www.starbucks.com/menu/product/424/iced?parent=%2Fdrinks%2Ffrappuccino-blended-beverages%2Fcoffee-frappuccino.

85 "Starbucks®." n.d. Accessed December 8, 2019. https://www.starbucks.com/menu/product/1033/single?parent=%2Ffood%2Fbakery%2Fcroissants.

86 Lobby, Mackenzie. "Avoid a Running Injury With the 10 Percent Rule." Active Network, LLC. 2019. Accessed November 2, 2019. www.active.com/running/articles/avoid-a-running-injury-with-the-10-percent-rule?page=1.

87 Hunter, MaryCarol R., Brenda W. Gillespie, and Sophie Yu-Pu Chen. "Urban Nature Experiences Reduce Stress in the Context of Daily Life Based on Salivary Biomarkers." Frontiers in Psychology 10 (2019). https://doi.org/10.3389/fpsyg.2019.00722.

88 Garlick, Peter J. "The Role of Leucine in the Regulation of Protein Metabolism." The Journal of Nutrition. 135(6): 1553S-1556S. June 2005. https://doi.org/10.1093/jn/135.6.1553S.

89 Leucine indirectly activates p70 S6 kinase as well as stimulates assembly of the eIF4F complex.
Kimball, Scot R., and Leonard S. Jefferson. "Signaling Pathways and Molecular Mechanisms through which Branched-Chain Amino Acids Mediate Translational Control of Protein Synthesis." The Journal of Nutrition. 136(1): 227S-231S. January 2006. https://doi.org/10.1093/jn/136.1.227S.

90 P70 S6 kinase has been shown to allow adaptive hypertrophy and recovery of rat muscle.
Bodine, Sue C., Trevor N. Stitt, Michael Gonzalez, et al. 2001. "Akt/mTOR Pathway is a Crucial Regulator of Skeletal Muscle Hypertrophy and Can Prevent Muscle Atrophy in Vivo." Nature Cell Biology. 3(11): 1014–19. 2001.https://doi.org/10.1038/ncb1101-1014.

91 Greenhaff, Paul L. "Creatine and Its Application as an Ergogenic Aid." International Journal of Sport Nutrition and Exercise Metabolism. 5(S1): S100-S110. 1995. https://doi.org/10.1123/ijsn.5.s1.s100.

92 Greenhaff, Paul L., Alice Casey, Anthony H. Short, et al. "Influence of Oral Creatine Supplementation of Muscle Torque during Repeated Bouts of Maximal Voluntary Exercise in Man." Clinical Science. 84(5): 565–71. 1993. https://doi.org/10.1042/cs0840565.

93 Kreider, Richard B., Charles Melton, Christopher J. Rasmussen, Michael Greenwood, Stacy Lancaster, Edward C. Cantler, Pervis Milnor, and Anthony L. Almada. 2003. "Long-Term Creatine Supplementation Does Not Significantly Affect Clinical Markers of Health in Athletes." Molecular and Cellular Biochemistry 244 (1–2): 95–104.

94 "Opinion of the Scientific Committee on Food on Safety Aspects of Creatine Supplementation." 2000. EUROPEAN COMMISSION HEALTH & CONSUMER PROTECTION DIRECTORATE-GENERAL. https://ec.europa.eu/food/sites/food/files/safety/docs/sci-com_scf_out70_en.pdf.

95 Poortmans, J. R., and M. Francaux. 1999. "Long-Term Oral Creatine Supplementation Does Not Impair Renal Function in Healthy Athletes." Medicine and Science in Sports and Exercise 31 (8): 1108–10. https://doi.org/10.1097/00005768-199908000-00005.

96 "Sleep Deprivation and Deficiency | National Heart, Lung, and Blood Institute (NHLBI)." Accessed November 3, 2019. https://www.nhlbi.nih.gov/health-topics/sleep-deprivation-and-deficiency.

97 Nedeltcheva, Arlet V., Jennifer M. Kilkus, Jacqueline Imperial, Dale A. Schoeller, and Plamen D. Penev. "Insufficient Sleep Undermines Dietary Efforts to Reduce Adiposity." Annals of Internal Medicine. 153 (7): 435–41. October 2010. https://doi.org/10.7326/0003-4819-153-7-201010050-00006.

98 NHLBI (n 94).

99 Mesarwi, Omar, Jan Polak, Jonathan Jun, and Vsevolod Y. Polotsky. "Sleep Disorders and the Development of Insulin Resistance and Obesity." Endocrinology and Metabolism Clinics of North America. 42(3): 617–34. September 2013. https://doi.org/10.1016/j.ecl.2013.05.001.

100 International Tables of Glycemic Index and Glycemic Load Values: 2008. [Table A1, A2] (n 49)

INDEX

Ab Roller, x
activity factor, 70–71
adaptive thermogenesis, 74–76
addiction
    to running, 235–236
    to sugar, 155–156
adenosine triphosphate (ATP), 90, 191, 195, 214, 216, 247, 266–267
age, and fitness, xii, 20, 33, 33–36
air displacement plethysmograph, 62–63
α-linolenic acid, 95
alcohol, 144–145
Alzheimer's disease, 137, 142–143, 234, 237
amino acids
    branched-chain (supplement), 113, 260–262
    essential, 93–94
    insulin and, 91
    whey protein powder and, 262–263
amyloid plaque, 143
Andretti, Mario, 247
android fat, 4, 63
anxiety, 38, 144, 147, 165–166, 235–237, 273, 290. *See also* mood
apps
    calorie counting, 84, 134
    for goals, reviewing, 14
    MyFitnessPal, 50–53, 83, 108, 133, 153
    Strong, 172
    for volume lifted, 174, 176
    for weight management, 62

Assaraf, John, 19
Atkins diet, x, 48
ATP (adenosine triphosphate), 90, 191, 195, 214, 216, 247, 266–267
Aurelius, Marcus, 17, 55, 217

back pain, 217–219, 222, 255
basal metabolic rate (BMR), 68–72
baseline, 68–72
BCAA (branched-chain amino acids), 113, 260–262
beauty standards, 5–6
before pictures, xi
Bellucci, Monica, 80
best version of yourself, 6, 34, 36
BIA scale, 60–62
bioelectrical impedance analysis (DSM-BIA), 60–62
blood sugar levels
    carbohydrates and, 90–93, 110, 264, 266
    sleep and, 275
    strength training and, 164
    sugar and, 139–141, 143, 147
BMR (basal metabolic rate), 68–72
Bod Pod, 62–63
body image, 165
bodybuilders, 30–31, 108, 123–128, 167, 267
bone density, 57–59, 63, 165
brain function, 137, 142–143, 234, 237
branched-chain amino acids (BCAA) supplements, 113, 260–262

bread, 142–144
bulking, 123–128
Burke, Edmund, 283

caloric deficit. *See also* macro/deficit split
    about, 45, 53
    calculating, 79–83, 85
    calorie counting and, 50–52
    calorie planning and, 52
    efficiency of, 45–46
    energy expenditure and, 67,
        71–72 (*See also* total
        daily energy expenditure
        (TDEE))
    exercise and, 49, 77, 239–240
    quantity vs quality, of calories,
        48–49
    science of, 46–47
    starvation for, 73–74
caloric density, 101–102
caloric expenditures, 67–72
calories
    cardio and, 240–242
    counting, 50–53, 84, 130, 145, 151
    daily number of, 7
    deficit of (*See* caloric deficit)
    densities, 101–102
    per fat pound, 78
    planning, 52
    surpluses, 47
cancer, 94, 97–98, 137–138, 167, 234
carbohydrates
    about, 89–90
    Alzheimer's disease and, 142–143
    caloric density of, 101–102
    consuming, timing of, 102–107,
        109–110, 112–115, 118–
        119, 121–122
    dietary guidelines for, 106
    energy and, 90
    foods with, 307–308
    glycemic index and, 92, 307–308
    gut bacteria and, 91–92
    insulin and, 91
    low diets of, 108
    as macronutrient, 88–89, 99
    powder (supplement), 263–266
    pros & cons, 92

    reputation of, 90
cardiovascular exercise
    caloric deficit and, 49, 77, 239–240
    calories burned during, 240–242
    fat loss and, 239–240
    health and, 234
    heart and lung health and, 233
    interval training and (*See* HIIT
        (high intensity interval
        training))
    joint health, 242
    macro split and, 110
    metabolism and, 235, 243
    mood and, 235–236
    muscular imbalance and, 243
    oxygen levels and, 234
    walking and, 253–255
    zones of, 244
cardiovascular health
    cardio exercises and, 233
    disease of, 4, 89
Carey, Drew, 151
casein (supplement), 146, 269–270
cellulose, 89
cheat eating, 83, 125, 134, 301. *See also*
    off-plan eating
chemicalories. *See under* food: fake
cholesterol, 89, 92, 98
classes (group fitness), 277–280
clean eating
    about, 129–131, 136
    filler ingredients, avoiding, 131–132
    strategies for, 132–135
Cohen, Alan, 223
collective acceptance, 5
competition
    benefits of, 278
    comparison to others and, 27–31
    and media's portrayal of fitness, 26
    social media and, 26–27
    subconscious, 27–29
compound exercises, 179–181, 185,
    207–208
Confucius, 197
control, of your mind, 34
cortisol, 254
creatine (supplement), 266–268
CrossFit, x, 49, 63, 132, 179, 278

cutting (for muscle maintenance),
125–128

dairy, 138, 145–146, 150, 269
data, of strength training gains. *See*
tracking strength training
gains
deficit. *See* caloric deficit
dementia, 137, 142–143, 234, 237
depression, 38, 144, 147, 165–166, 235–
237, 273, 290. *See also* mood
DEXA (also DXA) scan, 57–59
diabetes
carbohydrates and, 91–92, 141–142
cardio exercise and, 234
and fats, saturated, 96–98, 138
overfat and, 4–5
sleep and, 273, 275
*Dietary Reference Intakes: The
Essential Guide to Nutrient
Requirements* (Institute of
Medicine), 105–106
diets, fad, x, 48, 87
docosahexaenoic acid, 95
do-overs, infinite, 40
dopamine, 93, 154, 235
DORITOS 14
drug, food as a, 154–156
DSM-BIA (bioelectrical impedance
analysis), 60–62

eating clean. *See* clean eating
eccentric reps, 174, 177, 199, 201, 203,
211–213, 216
eicosapentaenoic acid, 95
embarrassment, xii, 51–52, 56–57
endorphins, 165, 235, 237
endurance, 192–193, 215
energy
adenosine triphosphate (ATP) and,
267
caloric deficits and, 53
carbohydrates and, 90, 92, 99,
104–105
expenditure (*See* total daily energy
expenditure (TDEE))
fats and, 95–96, 99
macro/deficit splits and, 121–122

metabolism and, 74, 78, 88
science of, 46–47
sleep and, 274, 276
strength training and, 191, 214
sugar and, 141, 147, 264
Epictetus, 129
exercise. *See* cardiovascular exercise;
exercises, for strength
training; strength training
exercises, for strength training
choosing, 179
compound, 179–181, 185, 207–208
essential, list of, 184–185
isolation, 181–184

fad diets, x, 48, 87
fake foods, 146–148
fast food, 14, 137–138, 242
fat burners (supplement), 270–271
fat calipers, 59–60, 65
fat loss. *See also* caloric deficit; macro/
deficit split
3- and 4-day splits for, 226–227,
229
cardio and, 239–240, 244–245
of large amount, 80–81
muscle building without, 123–126,
128
sleep and, 274–275
starvation and, 73–75
strength training and, 189–190
fat mass
about, 4, 69
calories and, 78
measuring (*See* measurement, of
body fat)
sleep and, 274
fats
about, 95–96
omega-3, 95–96
omega-6, 96
packaged foods and, 97
pros & cons of, 98
saturated, 94, 96–98, 106, 138
unsaturated, 96–97
filler ingredients, 131–132
fitness plans, 9–10, 291–293, 295–297,
299–301

flattery, xii, xiv, 23
food. *See also* food, and fat loss; food,
    limiting and avoiding
    fake, 146–148
    filler ingredients in, 131–132
    as fuel, 73, 88, 104–108
    junk, 131, 156–157, 243
    manufacturers, 156
    packaged, 97, 133, 148
    processed, 131–132
    quantity vs quality of, 48
    supply chain, 5, 97
food, and fat loss. *See also* food
    avoidance of (*See* food, limiting and
      avoiding)
    bulking and cutting, 123–128
    caloric expenditure and, 67–72
    cheating and (*See* off-plan eating)
    clean eating and, 129–136
    cutting and bulking, 123–128
    macro/deficit split and (*See* macro/
      deficit split)
    macronutrient balance (*See*
      macronutrient balance)
    macronutrients and, 87–89 (*See*
      also carbohydrates; fats;
      protein)
    through caloric deficits (*See* caloric
      deficit)
food, limiting and avoiding. *See also*
    food
    alcohol, 144–145, 150
    benefits of, 149
    dairy, 145–146, 150
    fake (with chemical ingredients),
      146–148, 150
    fast food, 137–138
    grains, refined, 141–144, 150
    sugars, added, 139–141, 150
The Food and Agriculture Organization
    of the United Nations, 7
form, for strength training
    about, 197–198
    drop sets and, 200–201
    focus on, 201
    help, seeking for, 202
    negative portion of reps, 201
    pace of, 199

    weight size and, 199–200
Frontiers in Public Health, 3
fuel, food as, 73, 88, 104–108

gadgets
    Ab Roller, x
    BIA scale, 60–62
    fancy bicycle, x
    kitchen scale, 51
Gandhi, Mahatma, 187
glucose, 90–93, 99, 164, 175, 235, 237,
    263–264, 266, 275–276, 307.
      See also glycemic index/load
glycemic index/load, 92, 141–143, 307.
      See also glucose
goal-setting
    about, 9–10
    celebrating, 11–12
    data for, tracking, 14–16
    small, 10–14, 16, 41
    thought process of, 12
    top of mind (*See* obsessive
      mindsets)
grains
    refined, 103, 141–144
    whole, 89, 103, 142, 150
greatness happens now, 9
groceries, 307–309
group fitness, 277–280
grouping exercises, 227
growth factor hormone, 235, 237
gut bacteria, 91–92
gym, dos and don'ts at, 283–286
gynoid fat, 63

heart health. *See* cardiovascular health
heart rates
    maximum, 244–245, 247–248,
      250–251
    target, 248
Hemsworth, Chris, 40
high-fructose corn syrup, 139, 150, 264
HIIT (high intensity interval training),
    247–251
hindsight, 34
histidine, 93
hormones
    amino acids and, 93

growth factor, 235, 237
hunger and, 76
insulin as, 91, 264
sleep and, 273–274, 276
and weight machines vs free
    weights, 183–184
Hugo, Victor, 101
hypertrophy, 190–192, 214

ideal bodies, 6
If It Fits Your Macros (IIFYM),
    111–113
Ildan, Mehmet Murat, 239
industrial food supply chain, 5, 97
inspiration, 29, 32
Instagram, vii, 26–27, 205, 284, 286
The Institute for Alternative Futures, 5
insulin, 91–92, 115, 149, 245, 264,
    274–275
isolation exercises, 179–182, 185
isoleucine, 93
Issawi, Charles, 259

joint health, 242
Jolley, Willie, 40
junk food, 131, 156–157, 243

Karnazes, Dean, 35
Katch-McArdle formula, 68–69, 72,
    289
kitchen scale, 51

LaLanne, Jack, 161
Laursen, Paul B., 3
lean body mass (LBM), 4, 69, 72
Lee, Bruce, 277
Lennington, Michael, 9
leucine, 93
lifting weights. See bodybuilding
Lima, Adriana, 80
α-linolenic acid, 95
Loeb, Allen, vii
lung health. See cardiovascular health
lysine, 93

macro/deficit split. See also
    macronutrient balance
    about, 115–116

caloric deficit, and training
    schedule, 116–118
caloric deficit, calculations of,
    119–121
and cardio exercises, 110
macro, and training schedule,
    118–119
macro, calculations of, 121
macro, determining, 107–111
macro, working vs resting, 106–107
macronutrient balance
    caloric density and, 101–102
    consumption schedule, 102–105
    daily percentages and, 105–107
    If It Fits Your Macros (IIFYM),
        111–113
    limiting, 103–104
    splits and (See macro/deficit split)
macronutrients, 87–89. See also
    carbohydrates; fats; macro/
    deficit split; macronutrient
    balance; proteins
Maffetone, Philip B., 3
man, on cliff, 28
Mansbach, Adam, 273
math, for fat loss and muscle gain
    calories and, 50–51, 83–84, 163, 241
    for fat loss, 47, 289–290
    off-plan and, 152–154, 157
maximum fat loss, 80
measurement, of body fat
    about, 55, 65
    bioelectrical impedance analysis,
        60–62
    Bod Pod, 62–64
    DEXA (Dual-Energy X-Ray
        Absorptiometry) scan,
        57–59, 64
    fat calipers, 59–60
    reluctance to, 56–57
media, fitness portrayal in, 5, 12, 26
mental health, 38, 144, 147, 165–166,
    235–237, 273, 290. See also
    mood
metabolic syndrome, 4, 243
metabolism
    bad food and, 149
    cardio exercise and, 243

clean eating and, 131
decreasing, 74–77
fad diets and, 46
genetic makeup and, 34
heart health and, 235
metabolic syndrome and, 4, 243
muscle growth and, 109, 124, 262
sleep and, 275–276
strength training and, 189
methionine, 93
metrics, for tracking strength training
    gains, 172
mindfulness. *See* visualization, positive
mindless eating, 6
mind-muscle connection, 205–209, 216,
    297, 303
mindset, of fat loss and muscle growth
age and, 33–36
competitive, 25–32
goals and, 9–16
obsessive, 17–24
overfat epidemic and, 3–7
setbacks and, 37–41
mobility, 165, 219, 228–229, 254
mood, 115–116, 144, 156, 165–166,
    235–237, 273, 290. *See also*
    mental health
Moran, Brian P., 9
Musashi, Miyamoto, 211
muscle
contraction, 206–207, 209
and cut phase for maintenance, 125
gaining, xvi, 19, 29, 33, 47, 110,
    123–124, 126–127, 190,
    229, 264, 290
imbalance, 243
metabolic effect of, 163–164
size, increasing, 190–192
MyFitnessPal, 50–53, 83, 108, 133, 153

nut flour, 143

obesity. *See* overfat epidemic
obsessive mindsets
about, 17–18
excessive, 20–21, 24, 76
tactics for, 22
through visualization (*See*

visualization, positive)
off-peak hours, 31
off-plan eating. *See also* cheat eating
about, 151–152
addictions and, 154–156
calorie tracking during, 153–154
cravings and, 156
as a decision, 152–153
eating disorders and, 157
scheduling, 156–157
omega-3 fats, 95–96, 309
omega-6 fats, 95–96
one-rep max, 176–177, 188, 214
overfat epidemic
calories and, 78
carbs and, 104
cause of, 5–7
data on, 3–5
sleep and, 275
overweight. *See* overfat epidemic
oxygen, 234, 237, 244, 247

P90X, x
packaged foods, 97, 133, 148
Paleo diet, 129–130, 142
personal trainers, x, xii, 168
perspective, 21, 47
pet peeves, gym, 283–286
phenylalanine, 93
Photoshop, 26
physics, 46
pictures, xi, 26
Pitt, Brad, 80
plans, 9–10, 291–293, 295–297,
    299–301. *See also* splits, for
    strength training
polysaccharides, 89
portion sizes, 5
positive visualization. *See* visualization,
    positive
preferred exercises, 184–187, 303–306
priorities, 79–83
problems, disappearing with fitness, 21
processed foods, 131–132
protein bars, ix, x, 148
proteins
benefits of, 93–94
as macronutrient, 93–95

pros & cons, 94–95
push *vs.* pull, 227

quantity *vs.* quality, of food, 48
quitting, and setbacks, 39

radiation, 57
Radiohead, 87
refined grains, 103, 141–144
reps
 drop sets, 200–201
 eccentric, 174, 177, 199, 201, 203,
   211–213, 216
 number of, 187–193
rest
 days, 223–224, 228
 of muscle groups, 225
 and sets, between, 214–215
restaurants, eating in, 132, 137–138
reverse pyramid, xiv
ripped, becoming, 23, 82, 250. *See also*
   under muscle: gaining
Rivera-Dominguez, Ivan, 3
roller coaster, of weight loss, ix, x
running addiction, 155–158

saturated fat, 94, 96–98, 106, 138
Schwarzenegger, Arnold, 80
secondary fitness goals, 109–111
The Secret, 18–20
Seneca, 3, 25, 33, 73, 233
setbacks, overcoming
 about, 37–38, 41
 inevitability of, 38–39
 moving forward from, 40
 as temporary, 39–40
shit happens, 38
single-digit body fat, 82
sleep, 273–276
small goals, 10–16, 41
snaccident, 123
Snickers candy bars, 14, 143, 264
social media, vii, 26–27, 32, 205, 284,
   286
splits, for strength training
 3- and 4-day, 226–227, 291–293,
   295–297
 5-day, 225–226, 299–301

building, 227
rest and, 223–225, 228
stages of life, 33. *See also* age, and fitness
Starbucks, 14, 242
starches, 89
starting point, 55–56
starvation, 69, 73–77
strangers, comparing yourself to, 26–27,
   29–30, 33–34
strength training
 about, 161–162
 approaches to, 187–195
 benefits of, 162–166
 carbohydrates and, 164
 effects of, 163–164
 exercise types of (*See* exercises, for
   strength training)
 form and (*See* form, for strength
   training)
 mind-muscle connection and, 205–
   209, 216, 297, 303
 myths of, 167–169
 rests and, 214–215, 223–225, 228
 splits for (*See* splits, for strength
   training)
 stretching and, 217–222
 tempo of, 174–175, 192, 211–214,
   216, 284
 tracking (*See* tracking strength
   training gains)
stretching, 217–222
Strong (app), 172
subcutaneous fat, 60–61
sugar. *See also* blood sugar levels
 added, 139–141
 addiction to, 155–156
 in alcohol, 144
 in dairy, 145
 fake, 147, 271
 grains and, 143–144
 metabolizing, 164–165
 monosaccharides and, 89
 saccharides and, 89
 synonyms for, 139–140
supersets, 193
supplements
 branched chain amino acid, 113,
   260–262

carb powder, 263–266
casein, 269–270
creatine, 266–268
fat burners, 270–271
vitamins and minerals, 268–269
whey protein powder, 262–263
sweets. *See* sugar

target heart rate, 248
TDEE (total daily energy expenditure).
    See total daily energy
    expenditure (TDEE)
tempo, training with, 174–175, 192,
    211–214, 216, 284
terminology, unintimidating, 4
testosterone, 33–34, 168, 183, 186, 227
theory of relativity, 46
threonine, 93
time under tension (TUT), 172, 174–
    177, 192, 203, 212–213, 216
top of mind, 23. *See also* obsessive
    mindsets
total daily energy expenditure (TDEE),
    45, 67–72, 289
total volume, 172–174, 176–177, 180–
    181, 192–193
tracking strength training gains
    data from, 171–172
    metrics for, 172
    one-rep max, 175–176
    time under tension (TUT), 174–
        175
    volume, 172–174
treadmills, x, 244
tryptophan, 93
TUT (time under tension). *See* time
    under tension (TUT)
12 Week Year, 9

*Ultramarathon Man: Confessions of an
    All-Night Runner* (Karnazes),
    35
unintimidating terminology, 4
unsaturated fats, 96–97

valine, 93
values, of macronutrients, 101, 118, 133
values story, 27–29
vegetarian diet, 94, 130, 267
visceral fat, 58–63, 65, 138, 167
visualization, positive
    about, 18–21
    examples of, 19–20
    of fat loss, 164
    power of, 29
    of results, 207–208
    setbacks and, 39
    time for, finding, 21–24
vitamins & minerals (supplement),
    268–269
VO2 max, 234, 237, 244, 247
volume
    total, 172–174, 176–177, 180–181,
        192–193
    and tracking strength training
        gains, 172–174
walking, 253–255
weightlifting. *See* bodybuilders; strength
    training
weight-loss roller coaster, ix, x
whey protein powder (supplement),
    262–263
whole grains, 89, 103, 142, 150
Whole30, 142

yo-yo effect, ix, x

zones, cardio, 244

ABOUT THE AUTHOR

Nate Clark is a writer, comedian, filmmaker, and fitness enthusiast. In addition to his original work for stage, television and film, he also directs commercials and industrial content for brands including Louis Vuitton, the New York Times, FENDI, Cartier, the Breeders' Cup, and many more.

He lives in West Hollywood, CA, with his husband and their son. And he used to be much fatter than he wanted to be.

Learn more at **nateclark.net**